Yoga *for the Young at Heart*

Yoga *for the Young at Heart*

Accessible Yoga for Every Body

Susan Winter Ward

Photographs by John Sirois

NATARAJ PUBLISHING

a division of

NEW WORLD LIBRARY
NOVATO, CALIFORNIA

Nataraj Publishing

a division of

New World Library
14 Pamaron Way
Novato, CA 94949

Cover and text design by Mary Ann Casler
Typography by Tona Pearce Myers

Portions of this book were previously published by Capra Press in 1994.

The material in this book is intended for education. No expressed or implied guarantee as to the effects of the use of the recommendations can be given nor liability taken. Please consult a qualified health care practitioner before beginning any exercise program.

Library of Congress Cataloging-in-Publication Data
Ward, Susan Winter.
   Yoga for the young at heart : accessible yoga for every body / Susan Winter Ward ; photography by John Sirois.
      p.   cm.
   ISBN 1-57731-222-8
   1. Yoga, Hatha. I. Title.
   RA781.7 .W369 2002
   613.7'046—dc21

2001008291

First Printing, April 2002
ISBN 1-57731-222-8
Printed in Canada on acid-free, partially recycled paper
Distributed to the trade by Publishers Group West

10 9 8 7 6 5 4 3 2 1

To the father/mother creator of us all
and
to my earthly creators,

my father, Carl, a sage and a saint,
and
my mother, Julia, my ally and an angel,

who both teach me about love,
confidence, patience, and trust.

Contents

When I was in college, my best friend told me about a practice she had discovered called hatha yoga. She thought I'd like it and urged me to try it. Thinking that it sounded like a healthy thing for my body, I enrolled in a yoga course. I soon discovered that yoga was indeed good for my body, and so much more — it contributed greatly to my emotional, mental, and spiritual well-being, too. In fact, I learned that hatha yoga is an ancient practice in which focusing on the body and breath helps us to become fully present with ourselves on all levels, and helps bring better awareness, balance, and harmony into our lives.

I enthusiastically described my experience of yoga to my mother, who at that time was a fifty-year-old professional woman leading a fairly sedentary life. She had also had back problems for many years and had found no effective help. She began studying and practicing hatha yoga, with wonderful results. Her back pain dissolved, never to reappear, and she felt healthier than she had in years. A few years later she retired from her career as a city planner and traveled to India, where she studied to be a yoga teacher. She spent the next fifteen years without a home, traveling the world teaching a very deeply conscious form of yoga.

It has been thirty some years since I first encountered yoga, and a simple hatha yoga practice is still an important part of my daily routine. I'm happy to say that my mother, now in her eighties, still practices yoga, swims in the ocean every day (she lives in Hawaii), and is in great health.

I hope this story will inspire anyone of any age who is curious to try hatha yoga. This book is a wonderful guide on that journey.

Shakti Gawain
author of *Creative Visualization* and *Living in the Light*
Mill Valley, California
February 6, 2002

Yoga is a gift in our lives, in fact one of the greatest gifts we have ever given ourselves. It has brought grace, strength, and flexibility to our bodies and allowed us to have greater agility in sports and in our pursuits in nature. Even more, yoga has become a way of being, a way of seeing, and a way of life.

In our years of being both students and teachers of yoga, we have witnessed exceptional transformations in people, some ever so subtle while some have been quite profound. It is no wonder yoga has been considered mysterious or dubbed "the fountain of youth," because its ability to restore the body and support the life force is quite magical, yet quite scientific, too. It begins with the first breath.

Most of us have never been trained to breathe properly. We considered it came as part of the package, and perhaps it did. But sitting in chairs and cars all day, living in congested cities, or watching the Dow rise and fall did not. These things throw our breath, our bodies, and our perspectives off. Learning how to breathe properly, to sit, stand, and walk, in essence how to live comfortably in our bodies, are areas that yoga and the practices in this book address.

The Flow Series, on which this book is based, was developed as a balanced daily workout. It uses the classical poses and breath work of hatha yoga and is designed as a moving meditation. The Flow Series combines body movements and breathing in synchronicity, creating strength and stamina, skeletal and muscular alignment, cardiovascular health, flexibility, and mental clarity. Allowing the mind to float upon the breath and the body to flow into the positions brings one increased vitality and creates a meditative state that can flow into daily life.

Susan Ward's keen appreciation of the benefits of yoga has been translated into her adaptation of the Flow Series into a yoga practice designed especially for the "young at heart." She has a strong compassion for beginners and for our older citizens and is committed to assisting them with their health and well-being through yoga.

The techniques in *Yoga for the Young at Heart* give you the keys to the benefits of a personal yoga practice. This series can be adjusted to each person's level and pace. All you need to do is begin. This book offers you both the beginning and the inspiration. We wish you a lifetime of living comfortably with your body and spirit.

Namaste.

Tracey Rich and Ganga White
White Lotus Foundation
Santa Barbara, California

Acknowledgments

Yoga has changed my life. When I took my first class, I definitely was not enthralled. But there was a little voice inside of me that said, "You don't have to like it, just do it." Experience has taught me to listen to and obey that voice. After my third yoga class I was hooked, and my body and soul would never be the same again. The experience just keeps unfolding in ever more surprising ways. The existence of this book in your hand is a perfect example.

This book seems to have been guided into reality. I never set out to write a yoga book, but all the pieces necessary for the creation of this work appeared at just the right time to indicate that it was to be written.

I deeply appreciate the privilege of being the one to bring it together and acknowledge with heartfelt gratitude all those who have participated in bringing it to all of us.

I would like to thank the following wonderful people in my life for their support and participation.

I am forever grateful to my dear friend, Star Riparetti, who dragged me to my first yoga class, and to my first yoga teachers, Ganga White and Tracey Rich, who have provided teaching and inspiration, the Flow Series and White Lotus retreats, to myself and so many thousands of others.

A special thank-you to my yoga teacher, John Friend, originator of Anusara Yoga, who guides me in the continuing expansion of my understanding and dedication to my yoga path.

I deeply appreciate and honor my dedicated senior yoga students, especially Babs Raymond and Evelyn Malcolm from my senior yoga class at The Samarkand in Santa Barbara; I've learned so much from them. Their positive attitudes and physical fitness are an inspiration to me and, I'm sure, to many others.

I never could thank my mother, Julia Winter Cohen, enough for all she's done for me all my life. So, in this case, I'll thank her from the bottom of my heart for being the catalyst that she is, and for her constant encouragement, support, and love.

Big hugs go to "my Sis," Maggie Sanders, the Colonel's daughter. She paved the way for me; pep talked me and started this ball rolling. My life would never have unfolded as it has without her love and example of an irrepressible Renaissance woman. I am forever grateful, inspired, and blessed.

This book wouldn't be complete without the photographic abilities, patience, and willingness of my buddy, John Sirois. Somehow we always seem to connect at special times in our lives to help each other out. This is most certainly one of those special times. And deep appreciation goes to the terrific subjects of John's photography: Otto Mortensen, Babs Raymond, Star Riparetti, Karl Schiffmann, and Anita Stith. They all cheerfully spent hours posing cooperatively for the photos and couldn't have been better models.

And for all of your support, love, and encouragement, thanks to Sharon and Kermit Case, Denise Rue-Pastin, Nancy Hewitt, Lora O'Connor, and Kevin Dalton.

Through this cocreative spirit, this book gives you the opportunity to begin to explore a new way of being in your body. It was written for you. May you use it in good health and enjoy the process of self-discovery and unfolding.

Yoga is an adventure. I have been continually impressed with the changes it makes in people's bodies and lives, including my own, and welcome you to your own personal practice.

Regardless of your age or physical condition, a gentle and consistent hatha yoga practice can be of significant benefit; in fact, it can change your life. The practice of hatha yoga builds strength, increases flexibility and circulation, and teaches deep relaxation through a series of slow and gentle body poses and controlled breathing techniques, which can be adapted to everyone's abilities.

This book can be your guide to developing a stronger and more vital body, regardless of your physical condition. All you need to reap the benefits of a yoga practice is a willingness to begin, and to be open to new ways of experiencing your body. Yoga is a process, not a goal. It is a continuing discovery of physical and psychological challenges met with gentleness and sensitivity through which your body may relax, open, come into balance, and become healthier. The yoga process opens us to greater awareness of our bodies and minds and sensitizes us to the inner voice of our spirits.

It's important to meet your inevitable resistances with gentleness and to encourage your body to relax. Mother Teresa has said, "Do no great things, but do small things with great love." So love yourself, listen carefully to what your body is telling you about its limitations, and respect it. In this way your yoga practice will be both enjoyable and beneficial.

This book is an introduction to yoga. If you should want to make an in-depth study of more of the yogic practices and traditions, I refer you to the hundreds of books that have been written on yoga and all of its attendant histories, philosophies, practices, and poses.

To make this little book concise and easy to slip into, I have kept it simple and to the point: to create a guide for a simple personal yoga practice specifically designed for *every body*.

It is presented in four sections, each focused on an aspect of the body, mind, and spirit. The "Yoga Practice" is a good, solid, basic beginning practice with a few additional poses for those wanting a bit more of a challenge.

"Embracing Menopause" focuses on addressing the body-mind-spirit interrelationships for those of us in that important life transition; but it is also supportive for women of any age.

Regardless of physical ability, we all benefit from the poses in the "Restorative Asanas" section, and all of us can find ways to integrate the "Sitting Fit" poses into our lives, share them with others, and bring more peace and harmony to ourselves and to our world.

The practice of yoga need not be intimidating for anyone, no matter what their physical capacities. As Ganga White of the White Lotus Foundation says, "Begin where you are and stay there."

We will begin with the basics: what is yoga and where did it come from?

Yoga

The origins of yoga are shrouded in the mists of time, but it is believed to have originated three to four thousand years ago in India. The first written summary of yoga was penned by Patanjali in about 250 B.C.E., but yoga was already thousands of years old then. Over the centuries, many theories, philosophies, and systems have developed as expressions of personal physical, spiritual, and mystical quests. Now, yoga classes of many different types and systems are popping up everywhere.

Traditionally, there are eight yoga paths, eight branches on the "yoga tree." Hatha yoga is one of them. Karma yoga is another. The Karma yogi seeks spiritual connection through work. Mother Teresa is a perfect example of a Karma yogini. Bhakti yoga is the path of devotion, and Jnana yoga is the path of knowledge and wisdom. The general term for the physical yoga path is hatha yoga. The purpose of hatha yoga was mastery of the body, in order to control it and allow the yoga practitioner to meditate for hours, even days, undisturbed by the physical vehicle. Today, there are as many different styles of teaching hatha yoga as there are teachers. When looking for a yoga teacher, don't be afraid to shop around until you find one who inspires you!

Yoga is not a religion; it embraces all philosophies and all religions. It's a personal practice, a personal path to inner peace, to maximizing your potential and connecting with your own inner guidance and personal power.

Hatha Yoga

The word *hatha* (pronounced HA-tah) comes from the Sanskrit *ha*, meaning sun, and *tha*, meaning moon. So, hatha expresses the balance of opposite forces, sun and moon, male and female, positive and negative. Yoga means union or reintegration. So in hatha yoga we have the union or reintegration of opposite forces. Through yoga, the mind and body can reintegrate and balance can be restored. The Buddha said, "To keep the body in good health is a duty, otherwise we shall not be able to keep our mind strong and clear." If our body and mind are balanced, strong, and clear, all other aspects of our world are open to us.

Flow Yoga

The concept of flow in hatha yoga is called "vinyasa." It relates to the linking of one pose to the next and to the next one and on and on. Ganga White and Tracey Rich, of the White Lotus Foundation in Santa Barbara, California, have developed the Flow Series, a strong and challenging yoga practice intended to build strength, flexibility, and stamina. The yoga practice developed in this book is an adaptation of their Flow Series and has been strongly influenced by John Friend's principles of alignment of Anusara Yoga.

It is designed to create the same type of benefits as a more vigorous practice, yet is adapted for those with less strength and athletic ability.

The vinyasa, or flow, style of yoga allows the body to flow gracefully from one pose into the next to create a peaceful moving meditation. The series of poses in this guidebook are meant to be linked together through the body and the breath moving in harmony. Rather than thinking of this practice as a set of separate poses, they are intended to be integrated from beginning to end and thought of as a continuous movement.

If the entire series seems too challenging to you, begin by briefly holding each pose and moving slowly from one pose into the next until that process becomes easier. Begin by holding the poses for a short time and gradually move toward smoothing out the transitions between poses and increasing your holding time.

Dedication

We all have heard that practice makes perfect, but in the case of a yoga practice, there is no perfection. The more consistent the practice, however, the more quickly the results will become evident. I've heard many new yoga students enthusiastically report that they felt relaxed, energized, and an inch taller after their first yoga class. Everyone's first yoga experience is a personal one, and the feelings and effects vary as one's practice unfolds. The results become more refined and subtle over time and remain forever powerful. A yoga practice is an ever-changing experience. Remember, today's practice will be different from tomorrow's; your right side is different from your left; and your body changes from one moment to the next. Constant open-mindedness and allowing your body to be just the way it is at each moment will create an atmosphere of relaxation and acceptance in every moment of your practice.

Begin slowly. You will discover how much time each week feels right for you. Consistency is important. It is better to do twenty minutes of yoga every day than two hours once a week. A balanced practice for one person may be one-and-a-half hours every other day; for another it may be a half hour every day. Throw away your rigid schedule, but be consistent. If you tune in and listen to your body, it will tell you what feels appropriate.

It also helps to note benchmarks of progression in your practice. For example, make a mental note that your hands come just below your knees in a forward fold. Several weeks later you may notice that your hands come to the center of your shins. It's exciting to be able to look back and see how your body has changed.

Attitude

Hatha yoga requires that you be ultimately responsible for your own health. Stiffness, poor circulation, digestive problems, lack of physical strength, and many other ailments do not need to be accepted as the inevitable results of aging. A consistent practice of yoga, along with a healthy diet and positive attitude, can relieve those and other symptoms commonly associated with the aging process. They can be replaced with increased flexibility, efficient circulation and digestion, and increased strength. Consistent yoga brings a sense of connection, well-being, and clarity, all of which allow life to be more dynamic and enjoyable.

Be kind and gentle with yourself. If this type of stretching and breathing is new to you, it will take time to get used to it and develop your awareness of what your body is telling you. Listen to your body; explore your limits and tensions gently. Go slowly, and always respect pain. If a pose is hurting you, stop, back off to the point of a comfortable stretch, breathe, and allow your body to release slowly. Remember, there is no goal: yoga is a lifelong learning process of personal unfoldment; it's getting to know yourself from the inside out.

How you approach your yoga practice, your priorities, patience, and sensitivity, can tell you quite a bit about how you approach life. I've found that how I approach my yoga practice is a microcosm of how I approach challenges, implement self-discipline, respond to discomfort, and integrate spirituality into my life. The personal lessons that we need to learn seem to be reflected in our yoga practice. Take the seat of the observer and watch yourself objectively. It's quite an interesting experience.

A Word about Diet

In caring for our bodies, it's important to be aware that they need nutritious and health-giving foods. Much of what is presented to us as food is convenient, nicely packaged, and/or highly processed. It is filled with additives, preservatives, and mostly devoid of nutritional value. The cumulative effects of chemicals, toxins, stress, and environmental hazards in our bodies cannot be measured and exist in different combinations unique to each of us. Awareness of the importance of nutritious eating, relaxation, and bringing our bodies into balance can help to cleanse us of these toxins.

Traditionally, yogis are vegetarians. Over the centuries they have found a vegetarian diet to be healthy, and many people practicing yoga find that eventually their taste for meat diminishes. Since there is now a body of evidence showing that many diseases commonly associated with aging can be prevented, alleviated, and possibly cured by eating a diet free of animal products and fats, this dietary alteration can have beneficial long-term effects. In the bibliography at the back of this book, you will find listed some of the many books on the subject. I encourage you to explore them. The consensus is that adding lots of fresh fruits and vegetables, whole grains and seeds, along with plenty of water, could be an extremely valuable alteration to your diet.

Breathing

The breath, or life force, is called "prana" (pronounced PRA-nah). We usually take our breathing for granted, but obviously we cannot survive for long without it. The prana, or breath, that we inhale brings oxygen and life force to every cell in our bodies. The way you breathe plays a key role in your yoga practice. By concentrating on the rhythm of the breath, the body and the breath harmonize into a flowing, energizing experience in movement.

Coordinating the breath with body movements allows the body to move more easily and can also control the intensity of the poses. Each pose is usually held for a period of three to five breaths (a breath is a full inhalation and complete exhalation). The poses then follow one after the other with the body moving in harmony with the inhalations and exhalations.

Try this example. Sit in an armless chair and inhale as you raise your arms out from your sides and overhead, then exhale as you lower your arms down by your sides. Experiment with this movement, first breathing passively and then intentionally, with your breath moving in harmony with your body. Do you feel the difference?

It may help to visualize for a moment what is actually happening when we breathe. Since we usually take breathing for granted, we don't realize what a miracle each breath is. The lungs are made up of millions of tiny air sacs that handle the exchange of gases in our bodies on the cellular level, cleansing and oxygenating the body. The lungs take up a considerable amount of space in the body, actually extending from the collarbones down almost to the bottom of the rib cage.

In general, we breathe shallowly, with only the top portions of our lungs. Experiment with the depth of your breathing by seeing how you can gradually bring your breath deeper into your lungs with each inhalation. Bring your breath gently into your lungs, imagining the expansion of each little air sac inside, as if you were inflating a myriad of tiny balloons.

It is also important to understand what is happening on a more visible level when we breathe. As air flows into the lungs during inhalation, the diaphragm drops, the rib cage expands outward and up, and the upper chest lifts. On exhalation, the diaphragm lifts, the rib cage contracts, and the upper chest drops.

Although this seems elementary, a way to get acquainted with this phenomenon is to place one hand at the arc of your rib cage over your stomach and the other on one side of your rib cage. As you inhale feel your stomach expand and your rib cage move outward. As you exhale, feel the contraction. Try this for a few breaths with your eyes closed to really experience what happens in your body when you breathe.

In order to keep awareness on the breath, yoga practice uses a breathing technique called "ujjayi" (pronounced oo-jai-ee), meaning "victorious." Using this technique, a sound is created similar to that of breathing through scuba equipment or a snorkel, or of a throaty snore. Hearing your inhalation and exhalation makes it easier to stay aware of your breath throughout the practice.

It can take a little practice to learn to make your breathing audible. The sound of the ujjayi breath comes from the soft palate at the back of the throat, almost like a purr or whisper. To learn this breathing technique, whisper the word *whisper*, prolonging the "-per" part as you inhale and exhale through your mouth several times. Concentrate on where the sound is coming from and continue the sound as you close your mouth and breathe through your nose. While practicing yoga, breathe only through your nose; the yogis say, "The mouth is for eating, the nose is for breathing." Try to keep your inhalations and exhalations of equal duration as you relax and listen to the sound of your breath. It may seem strange and awkward at first, but with just a little practice it will soon become a natural part of your yoga practice.

Breathing keeps your energy flowing throughout your body; holding your breath blocks that flow. Watch your breath. Your breathing rhythm is a clue as to how challenged you are. If you're holding your breath, if it becomes ragged, back off and breathe deeply. Practice your yoga at a level where you can maintain a consistent breathing pattern that's comfortable for you.

Relaxation

Allowing your body to ease into a pose is the key to a pleasant and effective yoga experience. If the body is pushed too far too fast, it will resist, as most of us do psychologically as well. If one has a mental concept of what the body *should* do and pushes it to achieve that concept, it is likely the body will experience tension, pain, and even injury.

Relax. Our bodies respond well to coaxing. If a pose initially seems too challenging, back away from the edge of your resistance, inhaling deeply; and then relax into the pose on the exhale. It's surprising how the body responds to the release of tension and to the relaxing sound of your breath. You will notice that the poses are active, not static, and that as your body releases, you can take the stretches a little further. The next time you do the same pose, you will notice how much more easily your body will be gently nudged into the stretch.

There is a particular type of relaxation in yoga practice called "savasana," and it is considered by many to be the big payoff. At the end of your yoga session, it is extremely important to allow your body to relax and integrate the benefits of your practice, and this form of relaxation is also very pleasurable, so don't miss it!

At the end of each session, lie quietly on your back, releasing your body weight to the floor. Take several long, deep, slow inhalations and exhalations and then allow your body to resume its natural breathing rhythm. Release all tension. It can help to visualize releasing tightness from your feet, ankles, calves, knees, and so on up through your body to the crown of your head. Allow yourself to completely relax for at least five minutes. It's just fine to fall asleep. You will arise from this deep relaxation with a renewed sense of well-being.

Where and When

Yoga time is your time; it is especially for yourself. Eliminate interruptions, unplug the telephone, turn off the TV, put the cat out, and clear your space of distractions. Yoga requires us to be attentive to our bodies and our breath. It helps to have a protective attitude about creating this time and space for yourself.

The best environment for yoga is one that is clean, free from drafts, and spacious enough for your body to move freely. A firm, nonslip floor surface like hardwood or a non-plushy carpet are preferable. Many people use a mat. If you do, be sure it is firm, nonslip, and that it is used on a firm floor.

Wear comfortable clothes that will easily move with your body. Avoid clothes that bunch up or are oversized. Dance tights, cotton pants, or shorts are fine.

Yoga is done barefooted. Socks allow your feet to slip around inside of them, and shoes interfere with the natural movement of the muscles of your feet. Give your body a break from restrictions, physical and mental!

Yoga is best done on an empty stomach. If you choose to do your practice during the day or in the evening, be sure to put two or more hours between your meal and your practice time, or between your yogurt and your yoga.

Choose a time of day that works for you, when you won't feel rushed or distracted. Some people rise at six A.M. full of vitality, and others don't come alive until ten o'clock at night. Although yoga can certainly get you going in the morning and relax you at night, let your body and your biological clock be your guides. The important thing is to be consistent in your dedication to yourself.

Resistance is natural. Sometimes the most difficult part of a yoga practice is getting started. Try telling yourself that you're going to do only the first six poses, then you'll find that it's feeling so good, it's no problem to continue. Try it, it works!

A Note of Caution

If you have any question as to the suitability of this practice for you or have any serious physical problems, have had recent surgery, or are suffering from glaucoma, high blood pressure, or hypertension, please consult with your physician before beginning this or any other exercise practice. It is especially important to check on the suitability of poses that require you to bend over forward or lower your head below your heart.

Reassurances

Whenever we try something new and different, it's natural to feel both psychological and physical resistance. Sometimes we begin a new experience or commitment with a burst of energy that soon fizzles. Yoga, however, is its own reward. Almost immediately, the body responds to the cleansing and oxygenating benefits of deep rhythmic breathing, and to the balance and increased efficiency of all the body's systems through the gentle stretching and relaxing into the poses. So be forewarned, yoga can be addictive. The body, mind, and soul love it!

Muscles that have been half asleep for years are about to be roused from their slumber and are bound to reawaken slowly. If you experience sore or aching muscles, a hot tub and/or gentle massage may help. Stretching the sore area very gently will usually bring relief.

There is a difference between pain and muscle soreness, and it is important to tune in to your body to distinguish between them. Pain is telling you that something is definitely wrong; you're pushing too hard or your body is out of alignment. Pain is your body telling you to stop immediately. Aching muscles are telling you that something is right! It can even feel good. You can feel the stretch of resistant places in your body, and you're challenging your body to become more flexible, stronger, and more vital. As you progress with your practice, your body may go through a process of realignment. Try not to let preliminary discomforts discourage you. The sure cure for them is to stay with a consistent yoga practice.

Don't be surprised if you feel new things happening in your body; it will be making changes as you progress in your practice. You are bound to feel different sensations as your body becomes more flexible, stronger, more relaxed, and your internal organs and systems come into balance.

You'll also notice how your approach to life changes. In retrospect you'll realize, subtly at first, that you're more centered, more relaxed, and have a more gentle and tolerant attitude as you go about your day: ah yes, the magic of yoga.

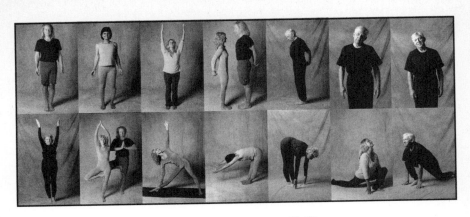

Welcome to Your
Yoga Practice

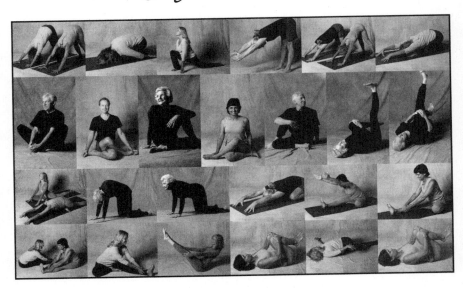

"The important thing is this: to be able to sacrifice at any moment what we are for what we could become."
— Charles DuBois

- ❖ Stand with the balls of your feet together and your heels slightly apart, arms relaxed at your sides.

- ❖ If helpful for balance, separate your feet hip width.

- ❖ Feel your weight evenly distributed on both feet.

- ❖ Press the soles of your feet into the floor as you lift through the crown of your head.

- ❖ Draw your inner thighs back and point your tailbone gently toward the floor.

- ❖ Lift your chest as you inhale deeply, drawing your shoulder blades onto your back and relaxing them downward.

- ❖ Draw the bottom edge of your shoulder blades forward, lifting your heart from your back body.

- ❖ Let your arms rest at your sides. Turn your palms to face outward and feel your shoulder blades against your back; hold them there as you relax your hands to face your thighs.

- ❖ Continue deep inhalations and complete exhalations, listening to the sound of your breath.

- ❖ Take five to ten deep and complete breaths.

- ❖ As you breathe, let your heart rise up and forward and extend through the crown of your head. Maintain the lift even as you exhale.

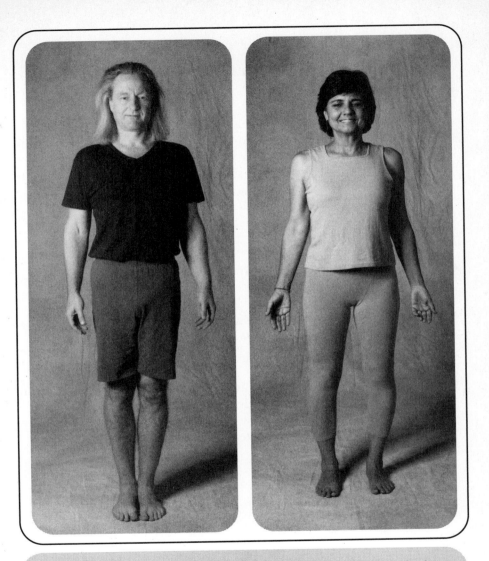

Benefits: Aligns body posture, evenly distributes weight on both feet, improves balance, and brings a sense of attentiveness and poise.

"The great thing in this world is not so much where we are, but in what direction we are moving." — Oliver Wendell Holmes

❖ Coming from the Standing Mountain pose, in the spirit of celebration, inhale, lift your heart, turn your hands to face outward, and raise your arms out from your sides, parallel to the floor. Then raise them all the way up and overhead, palms facing each other.

❖ As you lift, imagine pulling energy up through your feet; bring it up through your body and let it flow out of your fingertips.

❖ As you inhale, feel your ribs expand and separate as you lengthen your waist. Let your face shine upward.

❖ Maintain the lift as you exhale and stretch your fingertips toward the ceiling. Keep your shoulder blades flat against your back and your shoulders down.

❖ Keep your body active, energy moving all the way through your fingertips, lifting and expanding as you take three to five breaths.

❖ Moving into the next pose, take a deep inhalation and...

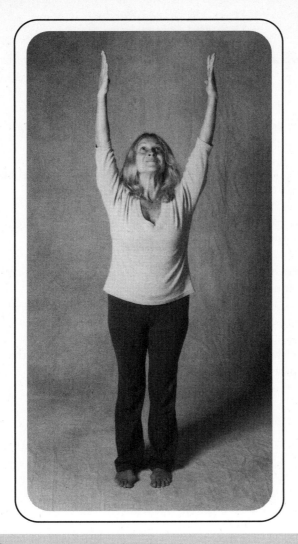

Benefits: Exercises the lungs and strengthens the muscles of the arms, shoulders, chest, and back. Stretches and tones the arm muscles, chest, shoulders, back, and abdomen. Strengthens posture and balance.

"It is the chiefest point of happiness that a man is willing to be what he is."
— Desiderius Erasmus

❖ Exhale as you press out through the heels of your hands and slowly lower your arms down to your sides.

❖ Press your shoulder blades flat against your back and clasp your hands behind you, elbows bent.

❖ Take a deep breath, and exhale completely as you press your knuckles toward the floor.

❖ Press your heart forward with your inhalation, and straighten your arms a bit as you exhale.

❖ Keep your chin pulled back toward your throat.

❖ Continue your deep breathing for three to five breaths. With hands still clasped behind you, move into the next pose...

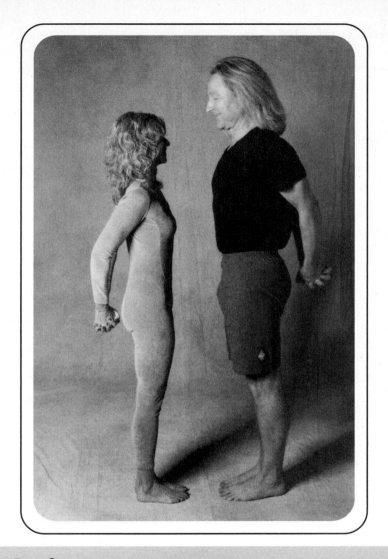

Benefits: Opens the chest and stretches and relaxes the shoulders.
Builds lung capacity, strengthens breathing, and stretches the abdomen.

"Whatever you can do, or dream you can, begin it! Boldness has genius, power, and magic in it."
— Goethe

Forward Stretch

❖ Keeping your hands clasped behind you, tuck your chin toward the soft spot of your throat.

❖ As you inhale, raise your chest toward your chin, expanding and lifting.

❖ As you exhale, gently bring your chin toward your chest.

❖ Bring your head forward until you feel a pleasant stretch down the back of your neck and between your shoulder blades.

❖ Breathe deeply. As you inhale, lift your chest toward your chin. As you exhale, soften your chin toward your chest.

❖ Allow the weight of your head to gently stretch the back of your neck and your upper spine.

❖ Relax into the stretch as you take three to five breaths.

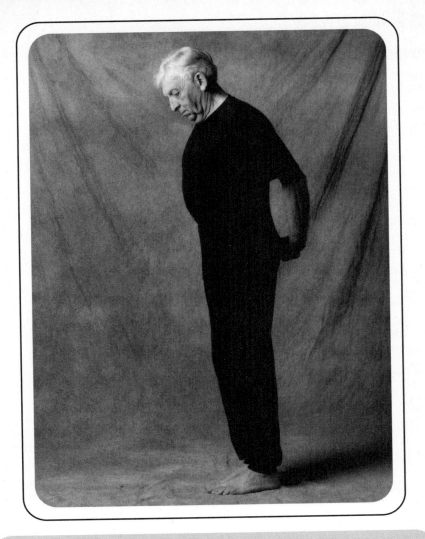

Benefits: Releases muscle tension in the back of the neck and upper back between the shoulder blades. Opens the chest and stretches the shoulders. Strengthens breathing.

Side Stretches

❖ Release your hands and allow your arms to be relaxed at your sides.

Right Side

❖ Keeping your chin tucked in, take a long, slow inhalation.

❖ Exhale as you tip your right ear toward your right shoulder; be sure your ear goes toward the shoulder, not your shoulder toward the ear.

❖ Keep your nose pointing straight ahead, allowing your chin to just slip to the left.

❖ Keep your shoulders relaxed, and gently press your left shoulder down as you exhale, releasing the left side of your neck.

❖ Take several breaths.

❖ Inhale as you bring your head back to center.

Left Side

❖ Keep your chin gently tucked in toward your throat.

❖ Repeat the stretch on the other side, bringing your left ear toward your left shoulder, pressing down the right shoulder as you exhale, stretching the right side of your neck.

❖ Remember to breathe deeply and give an equal number of breaths to each side.

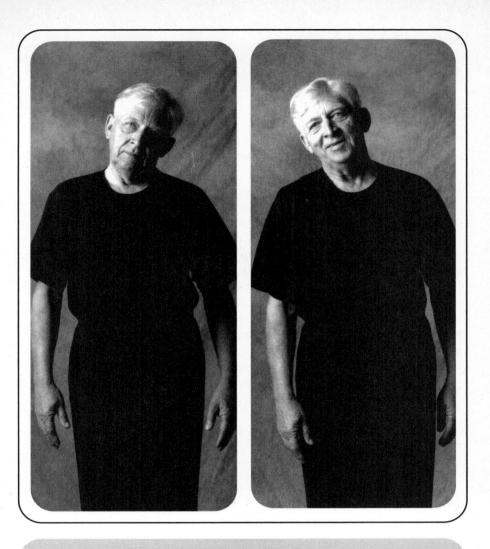

Benefits: Stretches and releases the sides of the neck and tops of the shoulders; strengthens the neck muscles.

"One can never consent to creep when one feels an impulse to soar."
— Helen Keller

❖ Stand tall with your heart lifted and the crown of your head reaching upward, arms relaxed at your sides.

❖ Rotate your palms to face outward and feel your shoulder blades come onto your back. Hold them flat as you take a long, slow breath.

❖ With your next inhalation, keep your heart lifting as you raise your arms out to the sides and overhead, palms facing up.

❖ Lift through your fingertips and press into the floor with your feet.

❖ Feel space being created between your ribs as you inhale.

❖ Maintain the lift as you turn your palms to face outward, press through the heels of your hands, fingers spread wide apart, and exhale as you slowly lower your arms.

❖ Take three to five breaths, then a deep inhalation as you move into the next pose.

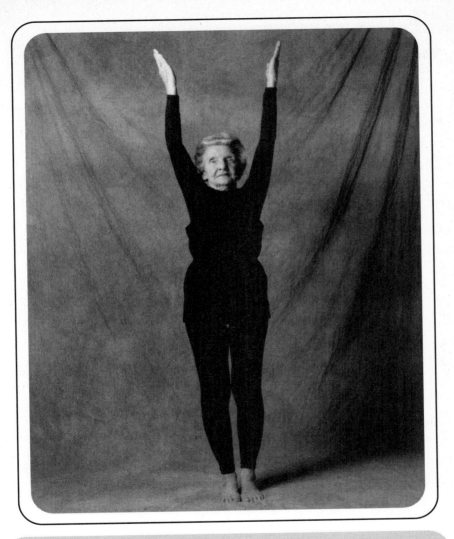

Benefits: Stretches and tones the arm muscles, chest, shoulders, back, and abdomen. Strengthens posture and balance. Exercises the lungs and strengthens the muscles of the arms, shoulders, chest, and back.

13

OPTIONAL POSE A: *Tree*

"Do what you can with what you have where you are."
— Theodore Roosevelt

❖ Stand squarely on both feet, lifting through the crown of your head.

❖ For balance, fix your gaze on a point in front of you.

❖ Bring your hands together in prayer position over your heart and inhale as you lift your right foot to rest against the inside of your left calf or thigh, your right knee pointing out to the right side.

❖ Breathe evenly, lifting through the crown of your head as you inhale. Press your standing foot into the floor as you exhale and hug your leg muscles to the bones. Be sure to keep your tailbone pointing down toward the floor to avoid unnecessary stress on your lower back.

❖ If you're feeling steady at this level of the pose, you may raise your arms out to the sides and bring your hands into prayer position overhead.

NOTE: If balance is challenging for you, you may begin practicing this pose with your hands on your hips, move to bringing your hands to prayer position over your heart, and gradually raise your arms overhead as you become more proficient.

❖ Repeat the pose on the opposite side.

❖ As you become more adept at balancing and more flexible, you may position your foot higher and higher against your standing leg.

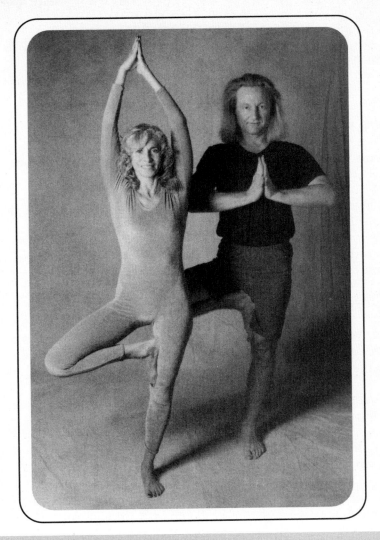

Benefits: Develops balance, concentration, and poise; strengthens buttocks, lower back, legs, feet, and ankles. Stretches ribs, shoulders, and arms.

"There is no failure except in no longer trying."

— Elbert Hubbard

❖ Step your right foot forward approximately 3 feet.

❖ Turn your back foot to a 90-degree angle, letting a line from the heel of your front foot bisect the arch of your back foot.

❖ Inhale as you raise your arms out to the sides, making sure that your hips are facing to your left.

❖ Your right hand reaches out toward your front foot and your back arm reaches over your back leg.

❖ Lift your heart and keep your shoulder blades against your back.

❖ Lift your torso from under your armpits, elongate the sides of your rib cage as you lengthen out of your hips and lean your torso to the right.

❖ Exhale as you lower your torso to the side, bringing your front hand toward your shin and raising your back arm up toward the ceiling.

❖ You may turn your head to look up at your raised hand or look down at your forward foot.

❖ Breathe deeply, extending your raised arm upward, extending forward through the crown of your head and back through your tailbone.

❖ Hold the pose and breathe. Take three to five breaths.

❖ Repeat on the opposite side.

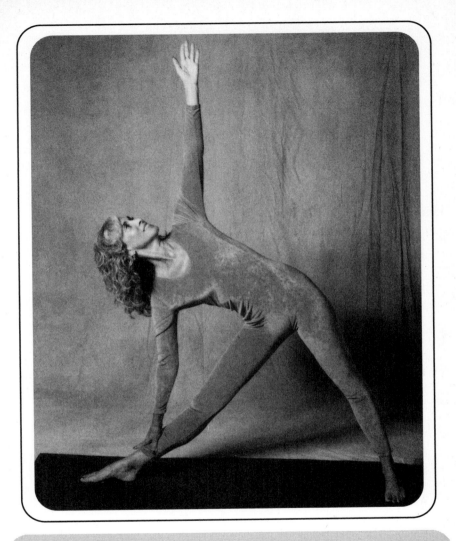

Benefits: Lengthens hamstrings, increases flexibility of the hips and spine, firms legs and waist, stretches arms, shoulders, and back, opens the chest, and nourishes the abdominal organs and spine.

"The thing always happens that you really believe in, and the belief in a thing makes it happen." — Frank Lloyd Wright

CAUTION: *This pose should not be attempted by those suffering from glaucoma, head injuries, high blood pressure, or hypertension without a doctor's permission.*

Moving from Tree or Triangle Pose...

❖ Stand tall with your feet parallel and planted firmly on the floor. Lengthen your spine and lift your heart.

❖ Keep your shoulder blades on your back as you raise your arms overhead and continue with the instructions below...

Moving from Pose 5, Arms Overhead

❖ Bring your arms out from your sides, level with your shoulders, and lead with your heart as you fold forward from the hips, exhaling slowly.

❖ You may keep your arms out to your sides, or extend them out in front of you. Be sensitive to the strength of your lower back and the flexibility of your hamstrings.

❖ As you come forward, keep your chin up and back flat as long as you comfortably can, then round over forward, continuing to roll down one vertebra at a time.

❖ If you feel any stress on your lower back, soften your knees.

continued

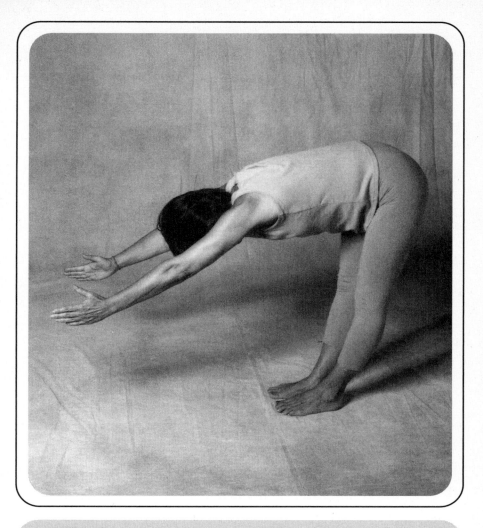

Benefits: Increases strength and flexibility of the spine and hips, lengthens hamstrings, and brings increased blood supply into the head and face. Massages the abdominal organs, relieves pelvic congestion, relaxes spinal nerves and the brain, and calms the nervous system.

- ❖ If you need to take several breaths, pause in your downward motion as you inhale, and then continue to roll down as you exhale.

- ❖ At the bottom of your forward fold, let your arms dangle toward the floor.

- ❖ Relax your neck and head, and then relax a bit more. We hold a lot of unconscious tension in our necks.

- ❖ Gently bring your breath as deeply into your lungs as possible and exhale completely. Take three to five breaths.

- ❖ Stay in this pose as you move into the next, the Arch . . .

Alternatives

If you have a weak lower back and the pose seems too challenging for you, you may want to experiment with some of these variations:

- ❖ Place your hands on your hips rather than bringing your arms out from your sides.

- ❖ Keep your knees slightly bent throughout the pose.

- ❖ Let your arms relax at your sides and roll down with knees bent and a rounded back.

If it is not safe for you to lower your head below your heart, you may try the following variation.

- ❖ Standing comfortably straight, inhale and extend your arms out to the sides at shoulder height, or place your hands on your hips.

❖ Exhale as you slowly come halfway forward, pivoting at the hip. Keep your chin up and your back flat.

❖ Inhale as you come up. Stay in this pose as you move into the next, the Arch . . .

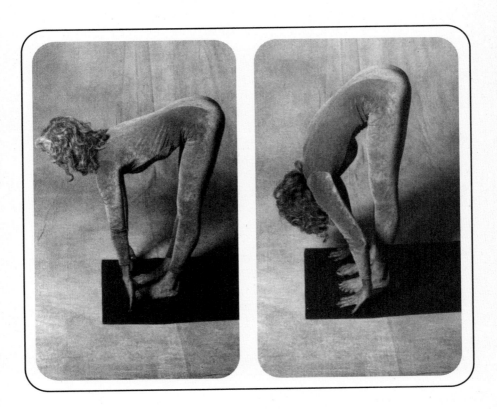

"Too much of a good thing is simply wonderful." — Liberace

❖ While still in the Forward Fold, allow your arms to hang relaxed or place your hands to the outside of your feet; if your fingers don't touch the floor, you may rest your hands against your shins or your thighs.

❖ Inhale as you arch up, pressing your chest forward and lifting your chin up. Let your heart soften toward the floor as your shoulder blades come toward each other on your back.

❖ Lengthen your spine by pressing out through the crown of your head in front of you and back through your tailbone behind you.

❖ Rotate your thighs toward the center line of your body and back behind you. Tune into the stretch in your sitting bones and hamstrings.

❖ Inhale as you arch up and exhale as you release back down into the Forward Fold.

❖ Repeat three to five times, and move into the Lunge...

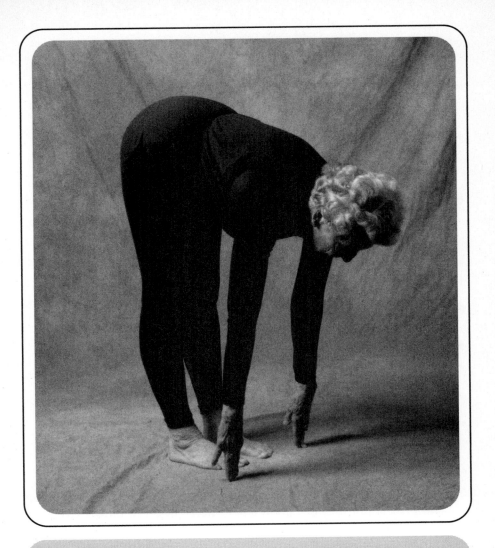

Benefits: Strengthens the back and increases spinal flexibility; tones the legs and lengthens the hamstrings, tones the nervous system, and stimulates the abdominal organs. Aids in digestion and elimination.

POSE 8: *Lunge (Right Side)*

"Do not be too squeamish and timid about your actions. All life is an experiment."
— Ralph Waldo Emerson

❖ Place your hands on the floor on both sides of your left foot and step back with your right foot. Bending your left knee, bring your hips toward the floor.

❖ Let your right knee rest on the floor and the front of your thigh face the floor; stretch your right leg back behind you as you inhale. Be sure that the top of your right foot is on the floor, with your toes pointing back behind you.

❖ Your left knee is bent in front of you and your front foot is flat on the floor. Imagine a straight line running along in front of your toes and fingertips.

❖ Let your fingertips touch the floor as you lift through the crown of your head. Breathe deeply and evenly for three to five breaths.

❖ Lift your chest away from your thigh as you gently stretch your right hip and thigh.

❖ Draw the energy from your back leg all the way up the front of your body and let it flow out through the crown of your head.

❖ Take a deep inhalation as you turn the toes of your right foot under and press them into the floor. Then, move into the Down Dog...

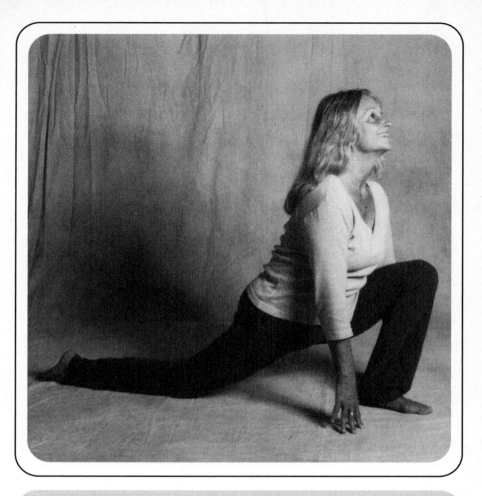

Benefits: Improves posture and balance, strengthens the spine, back, and legs, opens the hips, and tones the arms. Gives strength and flexibility to the legs, thighs, back, and abdomen; improves balance, and strengthens feet and ankles.

"Use your weaknesses; aspire to strength." — Sir Laurence Olivier

CAUTION: *This pose should not be attempted by those suffering from glaucoma, high blood pressure, or hypertension without a doctor's permission.*

❖ Exhale as you step your left foot back beside the right foot, which is behind you.

❖ Bring your knees to the floor and separate them hip width apart. Your wrists should be directly below your shoulders.

❖ Place the palms of your hands firmly on the floor, fingers spread wide apart. Soften your heart toward the floor and bring your shoulder blades toward each other on your back.

❖ Keeping your shoulder blades against your back, press the floor away from you with your hands and tip your tailbone upward, pressing your hips up and back behind you. Your body should form an upside-down V.

❖ Gently press your heels down toward the floor. If this hamstring stretch is too intense, try bending your knees, then straighten them gently one at a time.

❖ Tuck your chin softly toward your chest and try to keep your shoulder blades flat on your back as you lengthen your arms.

❖ Take three to five slow, steady, deep inhalations and exhalations.

NOTE: If you need to rest, you may come down to your knees, and bring your hips toward your heels. Remember to continue your ujjayi breathing, even when resting.

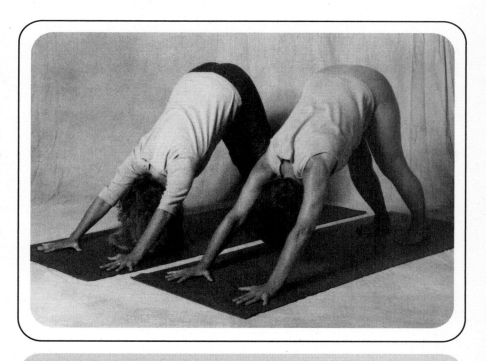

Benefits: Strengthens the upper body, stretches the hamstrings, strengthens the arms, legs, back, and shoulders, massages the abdominal organs, and tones the nervous and circulatory systems.

Alternative

If you are not permitted to do this pose for medical reasons, you may try the following variation.

❖ Come into the Child's pose by bringing your knees together on the floor and exhale as you lower your hips toward your heels. Keep your arms stretched out on the floor in front of you.

❖ To intensify the stretch, raise your palms and press your fingertips into the floor. As you exhale, walk your fingers forward. Hold the extension and keep your fingers pressing into the floor as you inhale. Be sure your hips and heels stay in contact.

❖ Let your head relax. As you inhale, feel the breath expand under your arms and release your lower back.

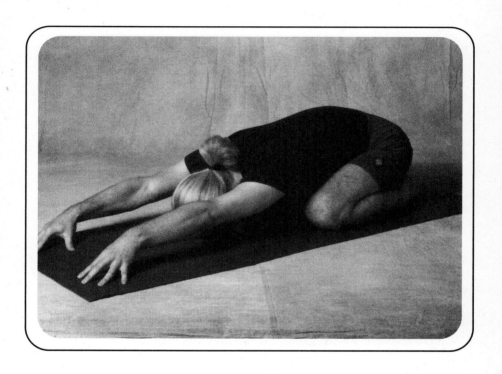

"What keeps the body restricted is not [always] a true physical block, but a mental pattern block. The blocks exist in the mind."

— Milton Trager

❖ From the previous Down Dog pose, inhale and bring your right foot forward, flat on the floor, between your hands.

❖ Exhale as you stretch your left leg out behind you, toes pointed away and the top of your foot on the floor.

❖ Inhale deeply again as you lift through the crown of your head. Come up onto your fingertips and lift your heart away from your right thigh.

❖ Remember to keep your heart lifted and your shoulder blades against your back as you breathe deeply.

❖ Feel the stretch in your left thigh and right hip.

❖ Keep breathing evenly for three to five breaths.

❖ Inhale as you bring your left foot forward to meet the right and relax into a Forward Fold.

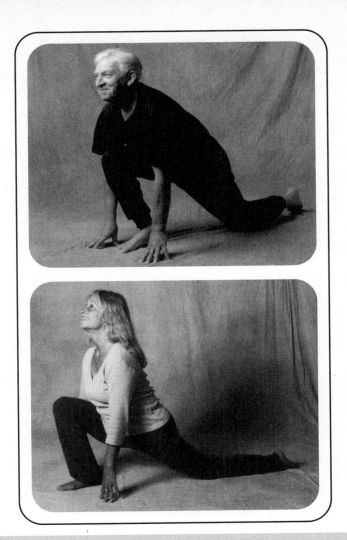

Benefits: Gives strength and flexibility to the legs, thighs, back, and abdomen; improves balance and strengthens feet and ankles. Improves posture and balance, strengthens the spine, back, and legs, opens the hips, and tones the arms.

31

"You gotta have a dream, if you don't have a dream, how you gonna make a dream come true?" — Rodgers and Hammerstein

CAUTION: *This pose should not be attempted by those suffering from glaucoma, high blood pressure, or hypertension without a doctor's permission.*

❖ Press into the floor with both feet, rolling inner thighs back and lifting your tailbone toward the ceiling.

❖ Exhale as you release your body forward and down into the Forward Fold.

❖ Keep your knees soft and go only as far forward as you can while keeping your knees straight.

❖ Roll your inner thighs toward each other and back again; feel the stretch in your hamstrings and the widening of your sitting bones.

❖ Take three to five breaths as you tune in to releasing and relaxing downward with each exhalation.

Alternative

If it is not safe for you to lower your head below your heart, you may try the following variation.

❖ Standing comfortably erect, inhale and extend your arms out to the sides at shoulder height.

❖ Exhale as you slowly come halfway forward, pivoting at the hips and keeping your chin lifted and your back flat.

❖ Reach out through the crown of your head and press back behind you through your tailbone. Inhale as you come up.

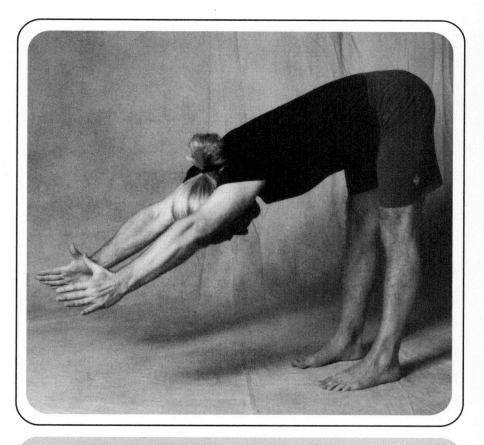

Benefits: Stretches the hamstrings and spine, firms and tones the abdominal organs and muscles, stimulates circulation, and brings increased blood supply to the head.

"Jonathan Seagull discovered that boredom, fear, and anger are the reasons that a gull's life is so short, and with these gone from his thought, he lived a long fine life indeed." — Richard Bach, *Jonathan Livingston Seagull*

CAUTION: *This pose should not be attempted by those suffering from glaucoma, high blood pressure, or hypertension without a doctor's permission.*

❖ If your hands touched the floor in the previous pose, the Forward Fold, you may simply place your hands on the floor beside your feet and step your feet back behind you to bring your body back into the upside-down V position, the Down Dog.

Otherwise:

❖ Bring one knee to the floor and the other down beside it.

❖ Position your knees hip width apart and directly below your hips; place your hands directly below your shoulders.

❖ Spread your fingers wide and press the palms of your hands flat against the floor.

❖ Keeping your arms straight, shrug your shoulders, soften your heart toward the floor, and bring your shoulder blades together flat onto your back.

❖ Let the front of your body soften toward the floor and let your back be concave.

continued

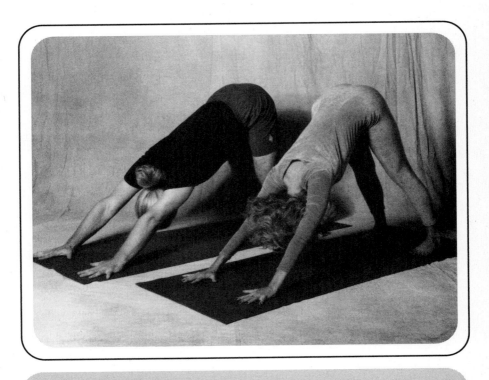

Benefits: Stretches the spine and hamstrings, strengthens the arms, shoulders, wrists, hands, legs, and back; massages the internal organs and increases circulation.

❖ Lift your tailbone upward and press your hips back behind you, pressing forward on the floor with your hands.

❖ Let your heels descend toward the floor and straighten your legs gently and slowly as you come into the Down Dog.

❖ Keep your chin toward your chest and your neck and shoulders relaxed as you continue to breathe deeply.

Alternative

If having your head below your heart is an issue for you, you may try the following variation.

❖ Bring your knees to the floor and exhale as you lower your hips toward your heels.

❖ Stretch your arms out on the floor in front of you.

❖ As you inhale, feel the breath expand under your arms and release your lower back.

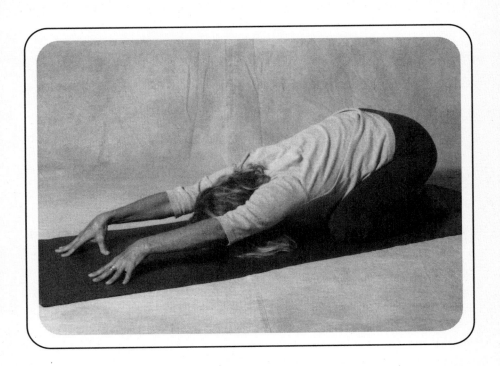

"Even if you're on the right track, you'll get run over if you just sit there."
— Will Rogers

Transitioning from the Down Dog position:

❖ Bring your right leg forward and lay it across in front of your torso, knee out to the right side, and slide your left leg back. You can begin with your right heel under your right buttock, and as you develop more flexibility, you can bring your foot forward and your knee out to the side.

❖ Stretch your left leg out behind you, as in the Lunge, with the top of your foot on the floor and your toes pointing away.

❖ Press your hands into the floor in front of you and walk your hands forward, stretching until your arms are outstretched on the floor. Breathe deeply for several breaths.

❖ Then, walking your hands back in, lift your heart up and forward, arching your back slightly and lifting through the crown of your head.

❖ Come up onto your fingertips and see how that creates space in the pose and allows you a deeper stretch.

❖ Breathe evenly, long, deep inhalations and exhalations for three to five breaths.

❖ Turn the toes of your back foot under and step your front foot behind you to meet your back foot. Come back into the Down Dog, pressing the floor away from you with your hands.

❖ Take several breaths, lengthening your spine.

❖ With an inhalation, bring the opposite leg forward to repeat the pose on the other side.

❖ Turn the toes of your back foot under and step your front foot back into the Down Dog, pressing the floor away from you with your hands.

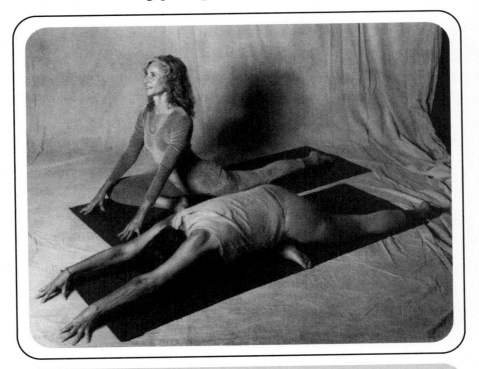

Benefits: Increases flexibility in the hips and groins, strengthens the back, opens the chest, expands the lungs, and tones the spine.

"The most minute transformation is like a pebble dropped into a still lake. The ripples spread out endlessly."
— Emmanuel, Pat Rodegast, and Judith Stanton

❖ From the Down Dog, come onto your knees. Make sure that your knees are directly below your hips and your hands are directly below your shoulders.

❖ Inhale deeply as you bend your elbows slightly and press your hands into the floor, bringing your heart forward and up between your arms.

❖ Press the crown of your head toward the ceiling and your tailbone upward, creating an exaggerated swayback.

❖ On exhalation, arch your back upward like a Halloween cat.

❖ Tuck your forehead toward your thighs, pulling your belly button in toward your spine.

❖ Repeat the movement several times, developing a smooth, flowing rhythm combining your movement and your breath.

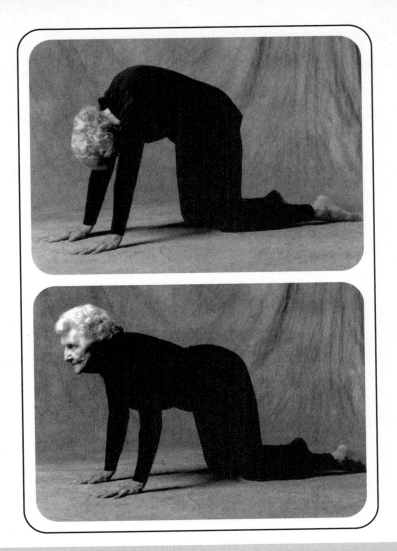

Benefits: Increases spinal flexibility, strengthens thighs, arms, and shoulders, tones the abdomen, and improves digestion, elimination, and circulation.

"The best pay for a lovely moment is to enjoy it." — Richard Bach

❖ After you've enjoyed the Cat Stretch, exhale as you bring your buttocks back toward or onto your heels.

❖ Inhale as you stretch your arms out on the floor in front of you, letting your head relax toward the floor. You may also try this pose with your arms at your sides.

❖ Breathe deeply; focus your breath, bringing it into your waist and expanding into your lower back.

❖ Feel the stretch in your armpits and the backs of your arms.

❖ To intensify the stretch, raise your palms and press your fingertips into the floor. As you exhale, walk your fingers forward. Hold the extension and keep your fingers pressing into the floor as you inhale. Be sure your hips and heels stay in contact.

❖ Feel your lower back release and your vertebrae separate as you breathe deeply.

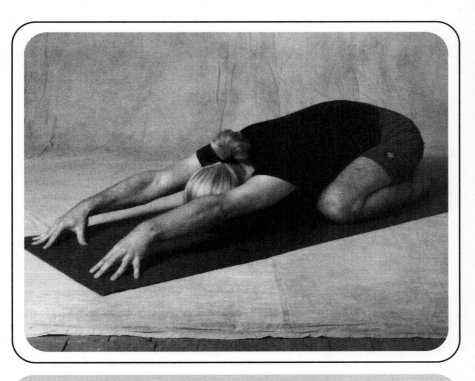

Benefits: Relaxes the spine, shoulders, and legs.
Stretches the rib cage, arms, shoulders, and neck.
Aids in digestion, circulation, and elimination.

"The greatest discovery of my generation is that a human being can alter his life by altering his attitudes of mind." — William James

❖ From the Embryo Stretch, sit up with your buttocks on your heels, then shift your weight to your left side, bringing your left hip to the floor.

❖ Your left knee will be bent in front of you. Move your right knee out to the right and bring the soles of your feet together.

❖ Bring your knees level with each other and balance your weight equally on your sitting bones.

❖ Let your knees relax out to the sides as you gently tip your pelvis forward, pressing your belly button forward toward your heels.

TIP: If it is difficult for you to sit up straight, fold several blankets and sit on them to raise your hips and release the tension on your hamstrings.

❖ Grasp your ankles with your hands and draw your elbows back toward your hipbones. Carefully flatten your back, keeping your shoulders relaxed and down.

❖ Lift through the crown of your head. Keep your elbows moving back and your heart moving forward.

❖ As your flexibility increases, you may tilt your torso forward, keeping your back flat and the front of your body lifting.

❖ Only go as far as you comfortably can; back away from the edge of the stretch, inhale, and soften into it with your exhalation.

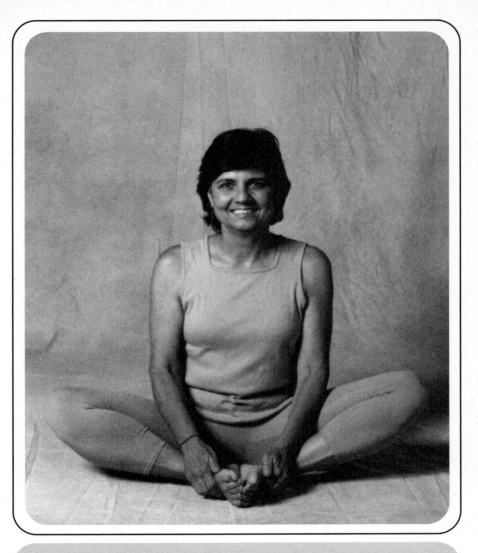

Benefits: Increases flexibility in the hips, strengthens the legs and lower back, and improves digestion and elimination.

"You can't build a reputation on what you're going to do."

— Henry Ford

❖ Extend your right leg out in front of you, keeping your left foot pressing lightly against the inside of your right thigh. With your hands, roll your inner thighs down toward the floor.

❖ Check that both hips are facing forward and that you are sitting squarely on your sitting bones.

❖ Maintaining a flat back, lift your heart, take a deep breath, and raise your arms up overhead, with your palms facing each other. Keep your shoulder blades against your back.

❖ With your next breath, lift out of your sitting bones and stretch up through the length of your torso, out through your fingertips.

❖ Press out through the heel of your extended foot, keeping your foot flexed, toes pulled back and heel pressing forward.

❖ Exhale slowly, coming forward carefully, leading with your heart, arms extended alongside your ears.

❖ When you've come to a comfortable level of stretch, let your hands grasp wherever they naturally come to rest without stress: your thigh, knee, shin, or foot. Remember to listen to the rhythm of your breathing, allowing your body to relax into the pose.

❖ Find the edge of the stretch, back away a bit as you inhale, soften into it as you exhale. Use your body and your breath together.

❖ Honor your limits.

continued

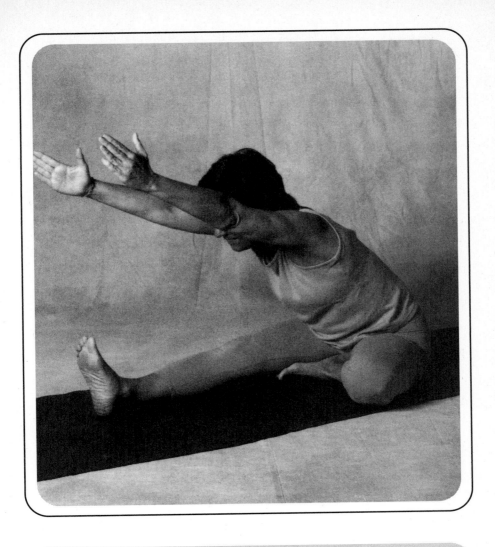

Benefits: Nourishes the spinal nerves and disks, stretches the hamstrings and ligaments of the back, tones the abdominal organs, and stimulates digestion and elimination.

❖ With each inhalation, feel your body open and expand, and with every exhalation, feel it release little by little, a breath at a time.

❖ Take five or more long, slow, even inhalations and exhalations.

❖ Bring your arms overhead and inhale as you come up with a flat back. Or you may slowly roll up as you inhale, allowing your hands to slide up your leg as you come to an upright, seated position. Exhale completely.

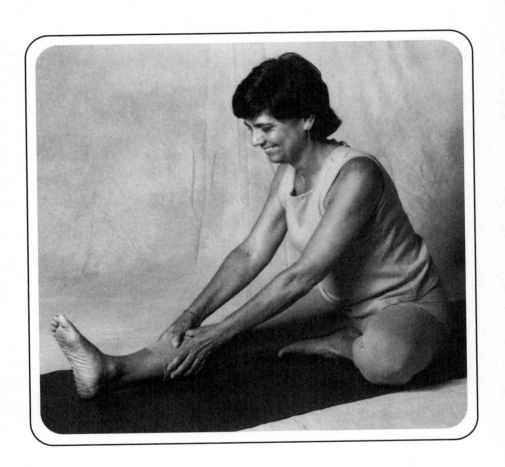

"Things won are done; joy's soul lies in the doing."
— Shakespeare, *Troilus and Cressida*

❖ Keeping your left knee bent, bring your right leg across to the left and rest it over your left leg.

❖ Bend your right knee and bring it onto the left so that the right knee is above the left.

❖ Let your feet rest alongside your hips and be sure that your heels are not resting under your hips.

❖ Lengthen your torso out of your hips; flatten your back and lift through the crown of your head. Keep your heart rising and your shoulder blades flat against your back.

❖ Let your hands rest on the soles of your feet or your knees and assume an air of nobility.

❖ If this pose is too much of a stretch, you may simply cross your right ankle over your left knee and allow your right knee to gently drop out to the side.

❖ Feel the stretch in your hips as you breathe deeply for three to five breaths.

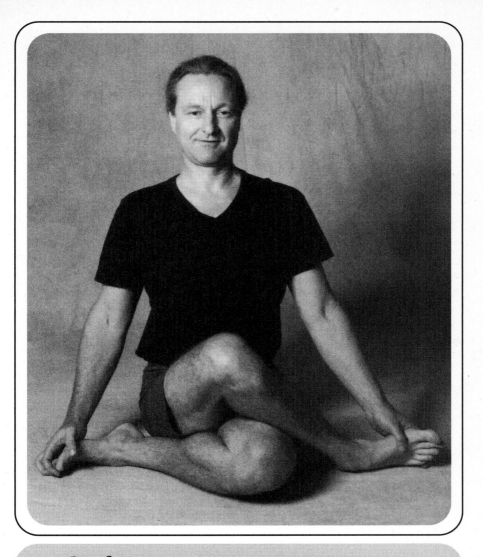

Benefits: Releases and strengthens the hips and lower back, stretches the ankles, opens the chest, and relaxes the shoulders.

"Stop chattering; go within."   — Sananda

❖ Place your right foot on the floor to the outside of your left thigh.

❖ Take a deep breath as you extend your left arm out to the side, shoulder height.

❖ Exhale as you bring it around your right knee, resting your knee in the crook of your elbow.

❖ With your next exhalation, bring the left side of your rib cage around a bit further toward your inner right thigh.

❖ Inhale as you flatten your back and raise your right arm up and overhead, lifting out of your hips and lengthening your spine.

❖ Exhaling, lower your right hand to the floor behind you, with the heel of your hand as close to your tailbone as possible, palm of your hand flat on the floor.

❖ Inhale as you lift through the crown of your head and exhale as you rotate your chin to look back over your right shoulder.

❖ Feel your spine lengthening with each inhalation and gently twist with each exhalation, using your front arm and leg as a point of leverage.

❖ Take three to five long, slow inhalations and exhalations.

❖ Come out of the pose gently. Inhale as you raise your right arm up overhead and exhale as you bring your body around to face forward again, lowering your arm.

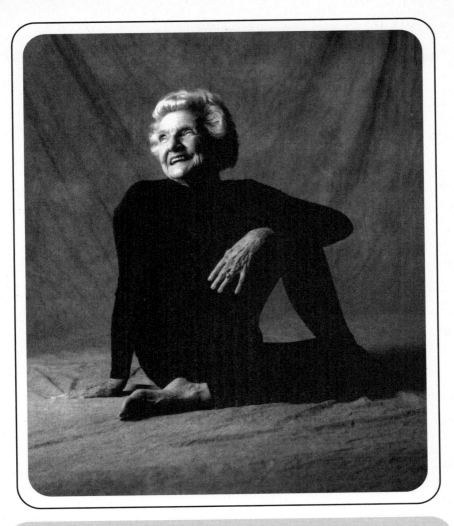

Benefits: Lubricates and nourishes the spinal column, increases elasticity of the muscles and ligaments of the spine, balances the nervous system; prevents backache, massages internal organs, toning liver, kidneys, and spleen. Aids digestion and elimination.

"You create your own reality every moment of your day."
— Shirley MacLaine

❖ Unwind from the Seated Spinal Twist and extend both legs out in front of you. "Walk" forward with your hips onto the front of your sitting bones and lengthen your spine.

❖ Press out through your heels, softening the backs of your knees to the floor.

TIP: If it is difficult for you to sit up straight with your legs extended, fold several blankets and sit on them to raise your hips and release the tension on your hamstrings.

❖ With your hands, rotate your thighs toward each other and down toward the floor.

❖ Inhaling, raise both arms out from your sides, then up and over-head, palms facing each other. Stretch up, separating your ribs, lengthening your waist, shoulder blades against your back.

❖ Exhale as you gently come forward, keeping your arms alongside your ears, shoulders back, and leading with your heart.

❖ Release your arms forward and let your hands come to rest on your legs, ankles, or feet. Keep your feet flexed, pressing out through your heels, and keep your heart moving forward.

❖ Breathe deeply for five or more breaths.

❖ Inhale and back away from the edge of your stretch, exhale and soften into the pose.

❖ Use your breath to release tension. Allow your body to slowly release tightness.

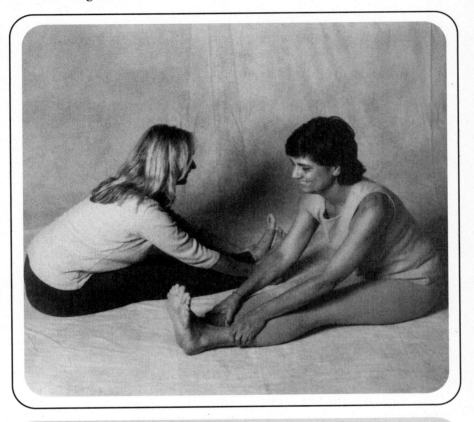

Benefits: Stretches the spine and hamstrings, increases circulation in the spine, and stimulates entire abdominal area as well as organs of digestion, elimination, and reproduction.

"All you can do is live as if your life depended on it. And watch what happens next." — Stephen Kravette

❖ Keep your left leg out in front of you.

❖ Bring your right foot in to press lightly against the inside of your left thigh.

❖ Be sure that your hips are facing squarely forward and that you are sitting up on your sitting bones.

❖ Rotate your inner left thigh down toward the floor.

❖ Take a deep inhalation and raise your arms out from your sides and overhead, palms facing each other. Lift your heart and press your shoulder blades onto your back. Lift up and extend your stretch all the way out through your fingertips.

❖ Keep your extended foot active by pressing out through your heel, toes pulled back.

❖ Exhale as you come forward slowly, keeping your back flat and leading with your heart. Extend your arms alongside your ears.

❖ Release your arms to their natural resting place, with your hands on your extended leg. If you feel stress in your lower back, lift your heart, flatten your back, and release the pose a bit.

❖ Listen to the rhythm of your breathing and use your breath to deepen the pose.

❖ Feel your body open up as you inhale and feel it release as you exhale.

❖ Take five or more deep, gentle inhalations and exhalations.

❖ Inhaling, come up with arms overhead and a flat back, or walk your hands up your leg slowly to come to a seated position.

❖ Exhale completely.

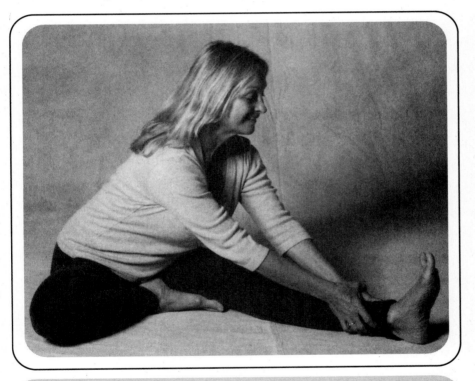

Benefits: Increases circulation in the nerves, disks, and muscles of the spine, massages the internal organs, and stimulates digestion and elimination.

"The first secret you should know about perfect health is that you have to choose it."
— Deepak Chopra

❖ Keep your right knee bent as you bring your left leg across and over your right.

❖ Bend your left knee and bring it around so that one knee is above the other. Let your feet rest beside your hips.

❖ Press your sitting bones into the floor, relax your shoulders, lift your heart, and extend through the crown of your head.

❖ Maintain a strong, flat back and let your hands rest on the soles of your feet.

❖ Feel the stretch in your hips as you lift your heart and expand your rib cage.

❖ If this stretch is too challenging, you may place your left ankle over your right knee and allow your left knee to drop gently out to the side.

❖ Breathe deeply for three to five breaths.

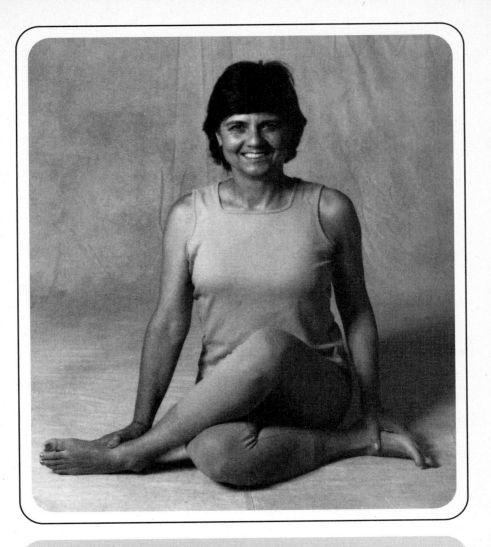

Benefits: Increases hip flexibility and strengthens lower back, stretches outer thighs, knees, and ankles, opens the chest, and relaxes the shoulders.

59

"Don't let life discourage you; everyone who got where he is had to begin where he was."
— Richard L. Evans

❖ Keeping your left knee bent, place your left foot on the floor to the outside of your right thigh.

❖ Inhale deeply as you extend your right arm out to the side, shoulder height.

❖ Exhaling, bring it around your left knee, holding your knee with the inside of your elbow. Draw the right side of your rib cage toward your inner left thigh.

❖ Inhale as you raise your left arm up and overhead. Keep your back flat and your heart lifted.

❖ Exhaling, lower your left hand to the floor behind you, as close to your tailbone as you can. Press the palm of your hand into the floor, lengthening your spine.

❖ Be sure that both sitting bones stay squarely on the floor.

❖ Inhale as you lift through the crown of your head and exhale as you rotate your chin to gaze over your left shoulder.

❖ Press against the floor to lengthen your spine with each inhalation and gently twist with each exhalation, using your front arm and leg as a point of leverage.

❖ Take three to five long, slow inhalations and exhalations.

❖ Come out of the pose gently, inhaling as you raise your left arm overhead and exhaling as you bring your body around to face forward again and lower your left arm.

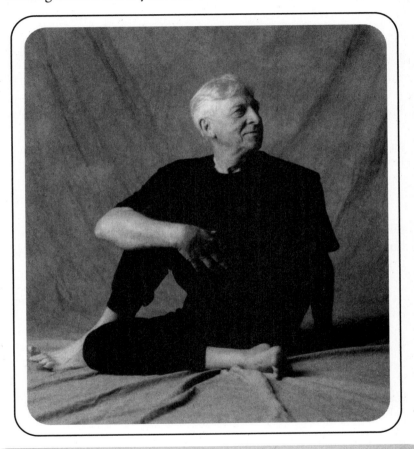

Benefits: Lubricates and nourishes the spinal column, increases elasticity of the muscles and ligaments of the spine, balances the nervous system; prevents backache, massages internal organs, toning liver, kidneys, and spleen. Aids digestion and elimination.

"There's only one corner of the universe you can be certain of improving, and that's your own self."   — Aldous Huxley

❖ Bring both legs in front of you, knees bent, balls of your feet on the floor.

❖ Hold your legs at the back of your thighs, just above your knees.

❖ Bring your shoulder blades together on your back, lifting your heart from the back of your body.

❖ Inhale as you lift your feet and draw your chest up and forward.

❖ Find your balance point as you tip back slightly on your sitting bones, slowly raising your shins. Keep your feet active, pressing out through the balls of your feet.

❖ Take a deep inhalation and exhale as you press out through the balls of your feet, extending your legs out in front of you.

❖ If straightening your legs is too challenging for you, keep your knees bent and, when you feel strong enough, straighten one leg at a time.

❖ Keep your shoulders relaxed and arms extended, either holding behind your knees or stretching your arms alongside your legs.

❖ Keep your chin down, your chest lifting, and feel your abdominal and thigh muscles supporting you.

❖ Maintain your deep breathing as you hold the pose for three to five breaths.

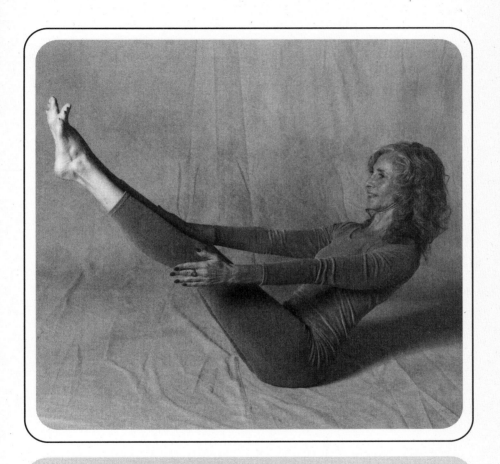

Benefits: Develops balance and strengthens abdominal muscles, thighs, hips, and back. Tones the nervous system.

"I take care of me. I'm the only one I've got."

— Groucho Marx

❖ Gently and slowly roll yourself back down to the floor, one vertebra at a time.

❖ Pull your knees into your chest.

❖ Place one hand on each knee and make circles with your knees together, first clockwise then counterclockwise.

❖ Smaller circles massage your lower back close to the spine and larger circles massage outward toward your hips.

❖ Experiment to see which feels best and enjoy your self-massage.

❖ Keep a conscious awareness of your breathing rhythm.

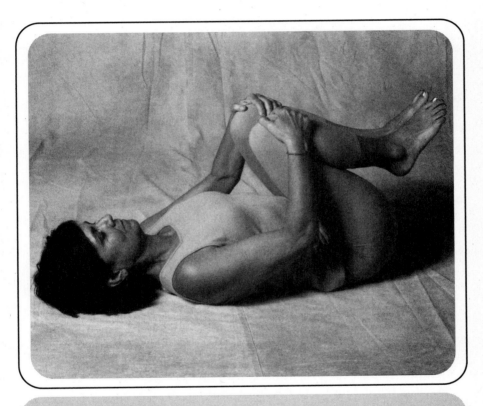

Benefits: A resting posture, it relieves lower back strain, massages abdominal wall and intestines, and relieves indigestion and gas pressure.

"Flow with whatever may happen and let your mind be free; stay centered by accepting whatever you are doing."
— Chuang-tzu

❖ Lying on your back, extend your arms out from your sides at shoulder level, palms facing the floor.

❖ Bend your left knee and bring your left foot to rest on top of your right thigh just above your knee or on your shin.

❖ Take a deep breath and press out through the heel of your extended right foot.

❖ Exhale as you lower your left knee across to your right side, bringing your right hand to gently press down on your left knee.

❖ Try to keep both shoulders against the floor.

❖ Inhale as you rotate your head to look toward your left hand. See if you can place your left ear on the floor.

❖ Exhale as you release your body into the pose.

❖ Continue breathing for three to five breaths, pressing out through your extended foot and releasing your left knee toward the floor.

❖ Take a deep inhalation and bring your left knee toward your chest. As you exhale, roll back to center.

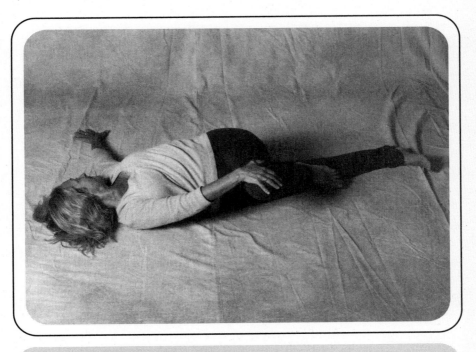

Benefits: Massages internal organs, stretches ligaments and muscles of the spine, increases spinal flexibility, and hydrates and nourishes spinal disks.

"There is nothing permanent except change." — Heraclitus

❖ With both hands, hold your left knee in toward your chest. Press out through the heel of your extended, right foot.

❖ Inhale and point the toes of your right foot as you squeeze your leg muscles to the bones and raise your right leg up toward the ceiling.

❖ Keep your right leg as straight as possible. If you feel any stress on your back, bend your knee a bit.

❖ Exhale as you flex your right foot and, leading with your heel, slowly lower your leg toward the floor.

❖ Point your toes and inhale, raising your right leg.

❖ Flex your foot and exhale, lowering your leg.

❖ Continue for three to five repetitions.

NOTE: If you would like more of a challenge, you may flex your right foot, press through your heel, and hold your extended leg a few inches above the floor for a breath or two before raising it again.

❖ Bring both knees into your chest.

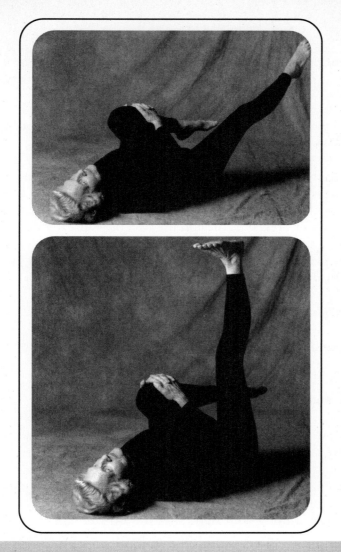

Benefits: Strengthens abdominal and lower back muscles and tones legs and hips.

POSE 27: *Lying Spinal Twist (Left)*

"A man consists of the faith that is in him. Whatever his faith, he is."
— Bhagavad Gita

❖ Extend your left leg out in front of you and your arms out from your sides at shoulder level.

❖ Bend your right knee and bring your right foot to rest on top of your left thigh just above your knee.

❖ Inhale as you press out through the heel of your extended, left leg.

❖ Exhaling, lower your right knee across to the left; gently press your right knee toward the floor with your left hand.

❖ Keep both shoulders against the floor.

❖ Inhale and turn your head to look over your right shoulder. See if you can place your right ear on the floor.

❖ Exhale and relax into the pose.

❖ Breathe evenly for three to five breaths, keeping your extended heel pressing away and your toes pulled back.

❖ Mentally direct your breath into resistant areas of your body.

❖ Inhale as you bring your right knee toward your chest.

❖ Exhale as you roll back to center.

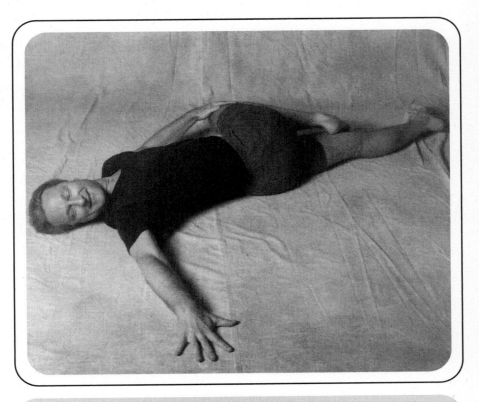

Benefits: Stretches, tones, and hydrates the spinal disks and ligaments, massages internal organs, and increases flexibility of the spine, back, and ribs.

"Do not look at your body as a stranger, but adopt a friendly approach towards it. To be sensitive is to be alive."
— Vanda Scaravelli, *Awakening the Spine*

❖ Lying on your back, hold your right knee in toward your chest with both hands and extend your left leg, pointing your toes.

❖ Inhale and raise your left leg upward, keeping your toes pointed and your leg as straight as possible.

❖ Flex your left foot and exhale as you press through your heel and slowly lower your leg to the floor.

❖ Point your toes and inhale, raising your leg.

❖ Flex your foot and exhale, extending out through your heel as you lower your leg.

❖ Continue for three to five repetitions.

❖ Bring both knees into your chest.

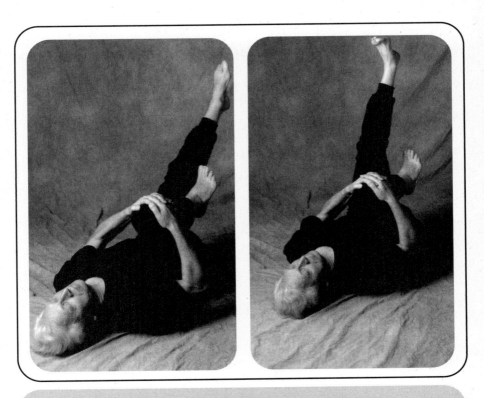

Benefits: Strengthens abdominal and lower back muscles;
tones legs and hips.

"Life just is. You have to flow with it. Give yourself to the moment. Let it happen."
— Jerry Brown

❖ Bring your knees into your chest. Place one hand on each knee.

❖ Circle your knees together to massage and relax your lower back.

❖ Circle clockwise and then counterclockwise.

❖ Breathe into your lower back as you release tension and increase circulation.

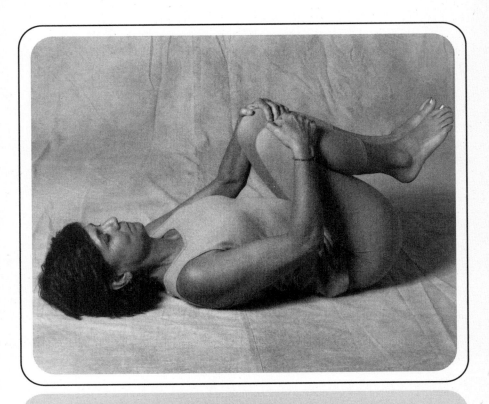

Benefits: Relieves lower back tension, massages lower back muscles and intestines, and relieves indigestion and gas pressure.

"It does not matter how slowly you go so long as you do not stop."

— Confucius

CAUTION: *This pose should not be attempted by those suffering from glaucoma, high blood pressure, or hypertension without a doctor's permission. If this is an issue for you, you may skip this pose.*

❖ Place your feet on the floor just in front of your buttocks.

❖ Roll your shoulders back and press your shoulder blades together to support your neck. Let your arms rest by your sides, palms down.

❖ Gently press the back of your head against the floor. The back of your neck should not be touching the floor.

❖ Inhale as you press into the floor with your feet and raise your pelvis upward, keeping your tailbone lengthening toward the back of your knees.

❖ Keeping your shoulders flat against the floor, clasp your hands together under your lower back and interlace your fingers. Straighten your arms.

❖ Breathe deeply and steadily, holding the pose for three to five breaths.

❖ Feel your buttocks supporting you from behind and your thighs holding the lift. If you feel you need extra support, release your hands and place them against your lower back.

❖ Take a deep inhalation and come up onto your toes.

❖ Bring your hands beside your hips, palms down, and exhale as you slowly roll down, one vertebra at a time, so that your tailbone touches the floor last.

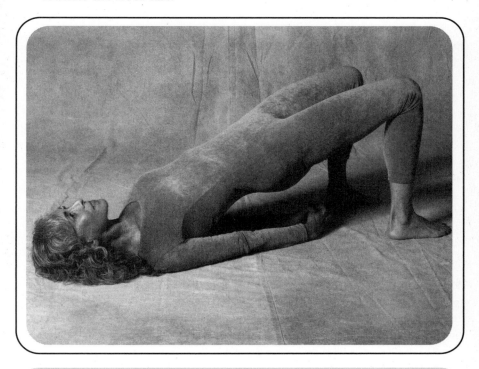

Benefits: Strengthens the buttocks, legs, and neck, increases flexibility in the spine, brings fresh blood to the head, opens the chest, and stimulates the pineal, pituitary, and thyroid glands.

"May you live all the days of your life."   — Jonathan Swift

❖ Lying on your back, raise your legs straight up, perpendicular to the floor.

❖ As you exhale, separate your legs into a wide angle.

❖ Press out through your heels and squeeze your leg muscles to the bones.

❖ You may support your legs by placing your hands on the outside of your thighs.

❖ Keep your breath even and hold the pose as long as is comfortable for you.

❖ You can come out of the pose either with straight legs or, if that is too much of a challenge, bend your knees and then draw your legs together, and bring your knees to your chest.

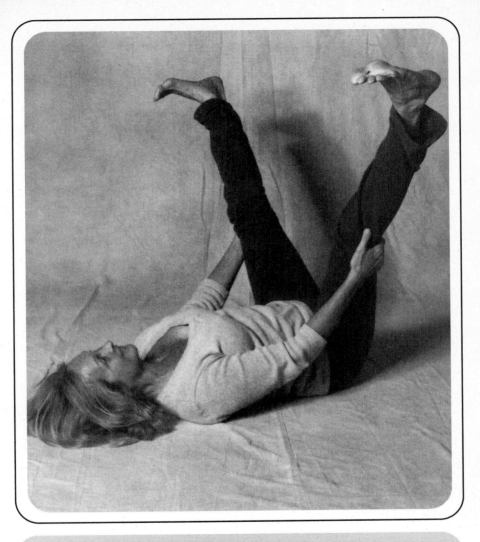

Benefits: Strengthens lower back, buttocks, and abdominal
muscles, stretches hamstrings, firms the legs,
and is beneficial for varicose veins and circulation.

"One is one's present self, what one was and what one will become, all at once."
— Peter Matthiessen

CAUTION: *Controlled breathing techniques should not be attempted by those suffering from glaucoma, high blood pressure, hypertension, heart, lung, or ear problems without a doctor's permission. If this is an issue for you, you may wish to skip this exercise.*

❖ Lying comfortably on your back, stretch your legs out on the floor in front of you and release your body to the floor.

❖ If you feel tension in your lower back, you may place a rolled blanket or a pillow under your knees.

❖ Take a long, slow, gentle inhalation while counting silently to five. Rather than forcefully sucking your breath in, invite your breath to fill your lungs. You are drawing in prana, the life force energy that infuses and animates everything in the universe.

❖ Fill your lungs completely and gently hold the air in for several counts.

❖ Exhale with control, counting to five as you exhale.

❖ Repeat for three to five inhalations and exhalations.

❖ Inhale slowly to the count of five, filling all the little air sacs, all the way to the bottom of your lungs.

❖ Fill your lungs completely, feeling your ribs expand and your diaphragm descend.

continued

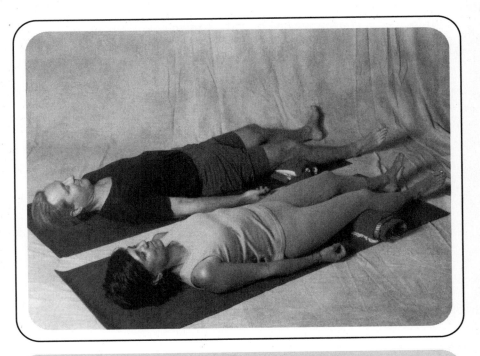

Benefits: Develops muscle control, increases lung capacity, produces a state of tranquillity, quiets the mind, detoxifies and oxygenates the body, lowers blood pressure, and triggers the parasympathetic nervous system into the relaxation response.

❖ Exhale entirely to the count of five, feeling your diaphragm lift as you release the air from your lungs.

❖ Hold your breath out for several counts.

❖ Inhale with control, again counting to five as you inhale.

❖ Repeat for three to five breaths, or for as long as you wish.

❖ Let your body resume its normal breathing rhythm.

NOTE: If it is too much of a challenge to breathe to the count of five, begin your breathing practice with counts of two or three and build up your breath control gradually.

Conversely, if breathing to the count of five is not challenging for you, increase your breath count gradually to build up your lung capacity and muscle control.

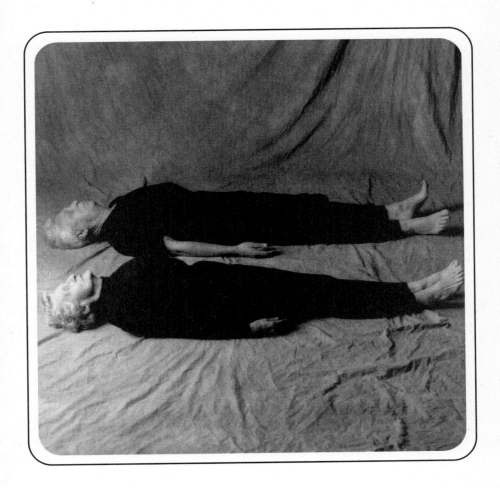

"My life has no purpose, no direction, no aim, no meaning, and yet, I'm happy. I can't figure it out. What am I doing right?"

— Charles M. Schulz

❖ Release your entire body to the support of the floor. Let your hands rest by your sides, palms facing up.

❖ Visualize each part of your body letting go as you mentally acknowledge your body from your toes up through the top of your head.

❖ Tell yourself to relax your feet and ankles, your calves and the back of your knees; release your thighs, lower back, and so on up through your body. Bring conscious relaxation all the way up to your jaw, forehead, scalp, and the crown of your head.

❖ Allow about ten minutes for this relaxation. This is an important time for the body to balance itself, gather energy, and integrate the benefits of your practice.

❖ It is very important to come out of the relaxation pose slowly to avoid dizziness or light-headedness. To come up, bring your knees into your chest and rest for a moment, then roll over onto your right side and remain in a fetal position for two or three breaths.

❖ Bring your left hand across in front of you and, pressing your hand into the floor, slowly unwind yourself up into a comfortable seated position with your eyes closed. Take five long, deep inhalations and exhalations.

❖ Thank your body for its service to you and thank yourself for caring for your body. Feel the benefits of your yoga practice, the sense of calm, centeredness, and relaxation, the vitality and strength and peace. Take that tranquillity, that peace, and share it in your world.

Namaste

"Namaste" is the traditional Sanskrit blessing spoken at the end of a yoga class. It means, "I honor the spirit of life, of truth, and of joy within you, and I honor that spirit within myself. When we acknowledge that we are both expressing that spirit, we are one."

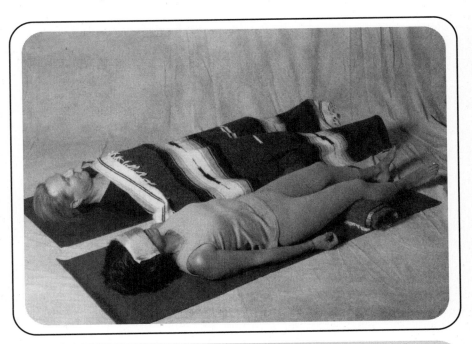

Benefits: Integrates the benefits of your yoga practice, induces the relaxation response, quiets the mind, reduces fatigue, and rejuvenates the body, mind, and spirit.

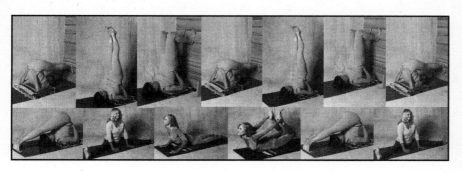

Embracing
Menopause

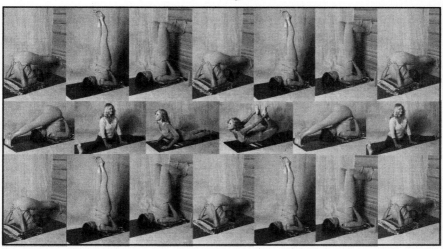

There are 45 million American women going through menopause. We can welcome and appreciate this special time for physical, emotional, and spiritual reassessment: by consciously embracing the menopause experience and deciding how we want to live the rest of our lives; by being responsible for how we choose to navigate this transition time; and by taking care of ourselves physically, emotionally, and spiritually. We can regard menopause as the opportunity for rejuvenation that it is and live more fully than ever with renewed vitality, inner peace, and power.

It is certainly a time when extra physical, psychological, and spiritual support are invaluable, and that support is available to us in the ageless art of yoga. Through yoga, we can balance our energies physically, emotionally, and spiritually. We can ease through our transitions naturally and gently phase into this new stage of our lives. Yoga soothes, balances, and rejuvenates all of the parts of us, bringing us to wholeness, allowing us to shine.

In addition to the Flow Series practice presented in this book, the following poses, along with the restorative poses described in the next section, can help to support and nurture you as you navigate the menopause years.

Caution: If you are having your period, inversions are not usually recommended. They increase the upward flow of energy in your body. The menstrual flow is a downward energy, so inversions are moving the energy against the natural flow at this time. Check in with your body, and if inverting feels good and appropriate for you, follow your body's lead.

"Attune yourself to personal energy, feel it flow like water, jagged stones of firm belief smoothed into nothing; cleansing, clearing, nurturing, healing. Follow it faithfully, honestly, spontaneously. Let it empower and serve."
— Haven Treviño, *The Tao of Healing*

CAUTION: *Inverted poses, like the Plough and Shoulder Stand, should not be attempted by those suffering from brain injury, glaucoma, high blood pressure, heart problems, or hypertension without a doctor's permission.*

❖ Place a folded blanket on the floor and lie on your back with the tops of your shoulders about 2 inches below the folded edge of the blanket. Position yourself so that the back of your neck does not touch the floor; if necessary, add another folded blanket to achieve the correct position.

❖ With your arms by your sides, roll your shoulders together behind you. Press your shoulder blades toward each other, creating support for your neck.

❖ Bring your knees into your chest and, pressing the floor with your arms, rock your hips toward your chin and lift your pelvis up, placing your hands on your back just above your waist to provide support.

❖ Extend your legs upward and then lower them toward your face until your toes touch the floor behind your head.

❖ Support your neck by gently pressing the back of your head into the floor, with your chin tipped slightly upward.

❖ Continue to breathe deeply. Stay in the pose for as long as it feels comfortable.

- ❖ From this pose you can go directly into the Supported Shoulder Stand.

- ❖ If you prefer to come out of the pose, bend your knees and bring your legs down slowly. Keep your knees tucked in toward your chest and roll to one side. Take a few deep breaths before sitting up.

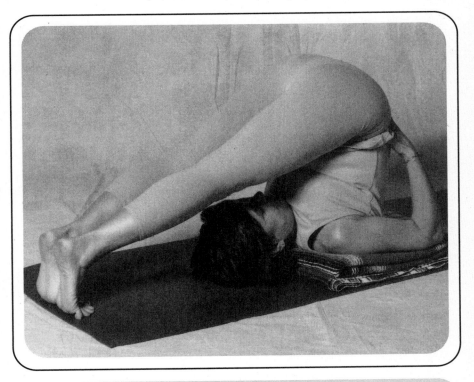

Benefits: Brings fresh blood to the spine and abdominal organs, relieves gas pains; weight bearing on the arms and hands helps to prevent osteoporosis, stiffness, and arthritis. Supports activity of the endocrine system, soothes the nervous system, and relieves headaches; stimulates the abdominal organs, relieves abdominal pain and bloat, releases toxins, and increases vitality — and much more.

Alternative

❖ Place one or two folded blankets under your shoulders and lie on your back so that the top of your head is about 18 inches from a wall.

❖ Set your shoulder blades flat against your back and shrug slightly.

❖ Bring your knees into your chest and, supporting your back with your hands, extend your feet toward the wall behind your head. Find your balance.

❖ Don't forget to breathe; stay in the pose for as long as you comfortably can.

❖ From this pose you can go directly into the next pose, the Supported Shoulder Stand.

❖ If, however, you want to come out of the pose, slowly bring your knees into your chest and roll to one side. Take a few deep breaths before sitting up.

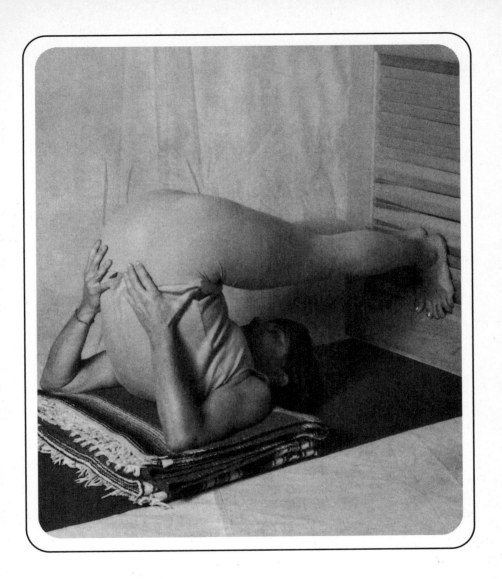

93

"No other stage of a woman's life provides as much potential for under-standing, plus the ability to tap into a woman's power, as does menopause."
— Christiane Northrup, *The Wisdom of Menopause*

❖ Place a folded blanket on the floor and lie on your back with the tops of your shoulders about 2 inches below the folded edge of the blanket. Position yourself so that the back of your neck does not touch the floor; if necessary, add another folded blanket to achieve the correct position.

❖ Coming from the Plough pose, set your elbows a bit wider than shoulder width and support your back with your hands at your waist. Slowly extend your legs upward.

❖ Bring your body into a vertical position, legs and ankles together, pressing out through your heels.

❖ Energize your legs by squeezing the muscles to the bones with a firm embrace.

❖ Keep your feet energized by pressing the balls of your feet upward and pulling your little toes back.

❖ Breathe deeply and stay in the pose for as long as you comfortably can.

❖ To come out of the pose, slowly bring your legs down, bending your knees if necessary and lowering your feet to the floor behind your head. Then roll down slowly, one vertebra at a time.

❖ Hug your knees to your chest for several breaths.

❖ Then roll onto your right side in a fetal position and breathe deeply before slowly sitting up.

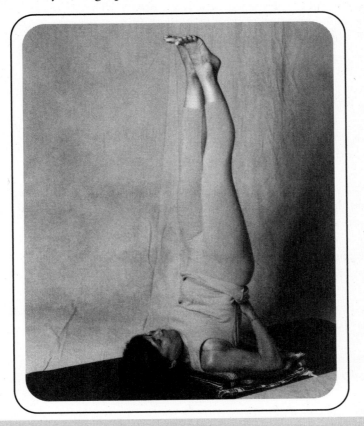

Benefits: Shoulder Stand is called the "queen of the asanas (poses)" owing to the multitude of benefits it brings: It balances the endocrine system, soothes the nervous system, lowers blood pressure, and relieves headaches; stimulates the abdominal organs, relieves abdominal pain and bloat, helps to prevent varicose veins, reduces swelling in the legs and feet, releases toxins and increases vitality, brings a sense of harmony and inner equanimity, and much, much more.

Alternative

❖ Place a folded blanket on the floor near a wall so that you will be able to lie on your back with your shoulders supported by the blanket, your head on the floor, and your buttocks touching the wall.

❖ Sit on the blanket with your left hip against or close to the wall. Pivot your body to the left and lie back on the blanket with your legs up the wall.

❖ Roll your shoulders together behind you. Press your shoulder blades toward each other, creating support for your neck.

❖ Bend your legs and place your feet on the wall, or you may slowly walk up the wall until you are inverted in a Supported Shoulder Stand against the wall.

❖ Support your waist by pressing your hands against your back, and straighten your legs as much as you comfortably can.

❖ Flex your feet by pressing upward through your heels and pulling your little toes back.

❖ Don't forget to breathe deeply. Stay in the pose for as long as is comfortably possible.

❖ To come out of the pose, slowly walk your feet down the wall, bring your knees into your chest, and lower your pelvis to the floor; keep your knees tucked as you roll onto one side.

❖ Be sure to take a few deep breaths before sitting up.

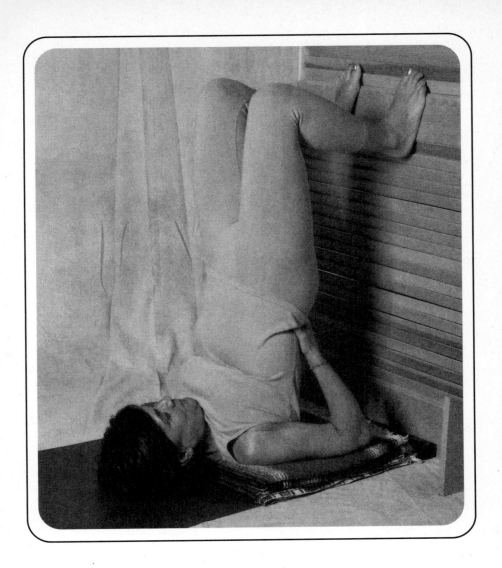

"Each woman is biochemically and spiritually unique. So is the hero's jour-ney that she must undertake if she is to succeed in her quest for wholeness."
— Leslie Kenton, *Passage to Power*

❖ Sit up straight and separate your legs to a comfortable stretch.

❖ Be sure that your legs are straight and your toes and kneecaps are facing upward. Using your hands, roll your inner thighs down toward the floor.

❖ Flex your feet and press out through your heels, keeping your legs straight. If this is a stretch for you, stay at this level of the pose.

❖ You may bring your hands to the floor behind your hips and press them into the floor to allow you to sit up straight. If you can main-tain the posture without the support of your hands, release them and rest them on the top of your thighs. If you have the flexibility, place your arms out in front of your thighs, with your palms on the floor.

❖ If you have the flexibility, while sitting up straight slowly and gently bring your heart forward, bending at the hips with your arms extended in front of you toward the floor. Keep your shoulders back and your back flat, with the front of your torso lifting. Lead with your heart.

❖ Find the edge of the stretch, take a deep breath, and back away slightly, then exhale and, maintaining the posture of the pose, soften into a comfortable level of the stretch.

❖ Use your body and your breath together to gently deepen the stretch.

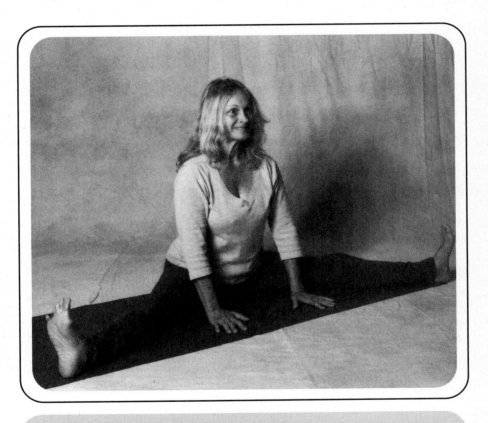

Benefits: Increases blood circulation in the pelvic area, stimulates the reproductive organs, and stretches hamstrings and lower back.

"When you sanctify your body-mind, you experience a sense of wholeness, a sense of power, strength, peace, knowing and gratitude. The power of life flowing through you spontaneously transforms you."
— Donald M. Epstein, *Healing Myths, Healing Magic*

❖ For this pose, you may want to use a blanket for cushioning under your abdomen.

❖ Lie on your belly. Place your hands flat on the floor under your shoulders, elbows tucked in beside your rib cage.

❖ Feel your feet, legs, and pelvis weighted against the floor.

❖ Keeping your shoulders back and slightly shrugged, press your hands into the floor and draw your chest forward and up.

❖ Press your shoulder blades against your back and push your hands down into the floor as you lift your chest and ribs.

❖ Keep your chin tucked back toward your throat and lengthen through the crown of your head.

❖ Lengthen your body with each inhalation and press your chest forward with each exhalation.

❖ Breathe deeply.

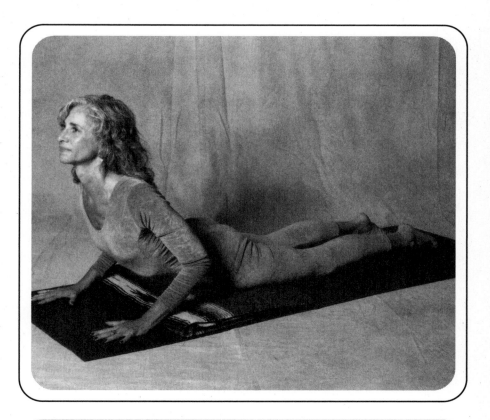

Benefits: Opens the front of the body; the pressure of the floor against the abdominal area stimulates and stretches, increasing circulation. Strengthens the upper body, develops flexibility and circulation in the spine, stimulates the adrenal glands, opens the chest, and expands the lungs. Helps to relieve lower back pain and digestive problems.

"It is essential to claim 'the pause' and find this new source of aliveness and meaning that will make the years ahead even more precious than those past."
— Gail Sheehy, *The Silent Passage*

❖ Using a blanket for cushioning, lie on your stomach and stretch your legs straight out behind you.

❖ Rest your chin on the floor and bend your knees, bringing your heels in toward your buttocks.

❖ Reach back and grasp both feet or ankles.

❖ Take a deep breath and raise your feet and your shoulders at the same time.

❖ Gently pull your feet toward your shoulders and press them upward as you raise your shoulders. Lift your chest away from the floor. Allow your legs to separate to give you more flexibility.

❖ Breathe deeply, stretching as gently and as fully as possible.

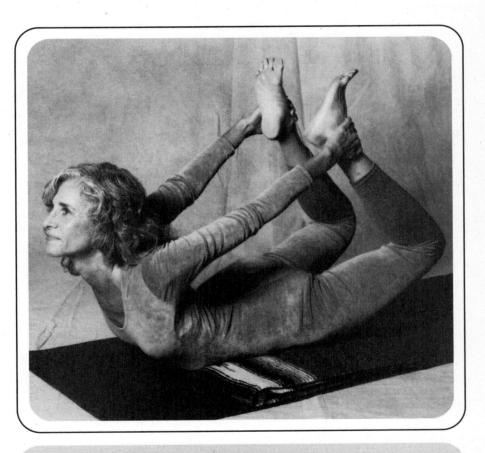

Benefits: Increases spinal flexibility and circulation to the cervical disks; also stimulates circulation of cerebrospinal fluid. Tones the abdominal organs, stimulates reproductive organs, and stretches and strengthens back and thighs.

"And so my empowerment becomes your empowerment and yours becomes another's. From a single light, all lamps may be lit. But there is more than a single lamp burning, there are hundreds of thousands of lamps burning on the planet. The way is well lit for those who are seeking it."
— Paul Ferrini, *The Ecstatic Moment*

❖ Lie on your back and bring your knees into your chest.

❖ Extend your arms out from your sides, shoulder level, palms facing the floor.

❖ Keep both shoulders on the floor throughout the pose.

❖ Take a deep breath. As you exhale, lower your knees toward your right elbow, keeping both knees tucked up and both shoulders on the floor.

❖ Turn your head to look at your left hand. Take several long, deep, full breaths.

❖ Feel where your breath goes in your body. Feel how the pose changes slightly with each breath, energizing and releasing tightness and tension.

❖ Inhale as you bring your legs back to center.

❖ Repeat on the other side.

The following poses are also suggested: Down Dog (pose 9, page 26), Forward Fold (pose 11, page 32), Cobbler (pose 15, page 44), Lying

Spinal Twist (poses 25, 27, pages 66, 70), and Leg Raises (poses 26, 28, pages 68, 72).

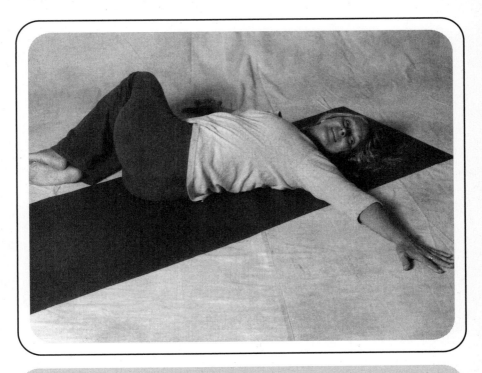

Benefits: Tones and stimulates the abdominal organs, strengthens the intestines and the abdominal wall, and relieves pelvic congestion; releases stiffness in hips, waist, and lower back.

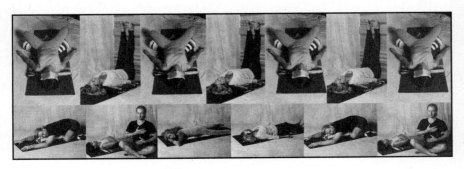

Restorative
Asanas

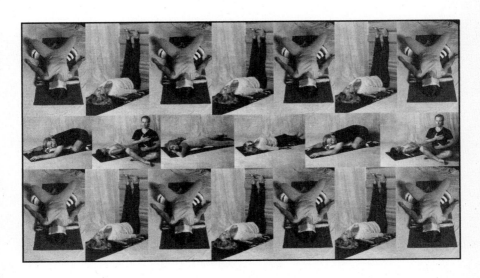

It's a crazy world. Not only does it seem to be spinning faster and faster, but we're also constantly dealing with stresses that are foreign to our bodies and minds. Nature didn't wire us to take in the amounts and types of stimuli that we're exposed to daily: microwaves, cell phones, toxins in our air, water, and food, traffic, violence — the list could go on and on.

How can we protect ourselves and find peace and harmony? Although we're dealing with pressures the ancient yogis never conceived of, yoga gives us tools that work.

Just a few poses can dramatically shift the energy of the moment from craziness to calm, from perturbation to peace.

We get so accustomed to daily tension that many times we don't even realize we're anxious. Our consciousness rides on our breath. By noticing the rhythm of our breathing, we can become aware of when we need to slow down, take time to breathe deeply, and bring ourselves back to a place of inner serenity. Our bodies take the signal from our breath; if we consciously slow it down, we relax.

The following yoga asanas (poses) can help you to come back to center. Set the mood for yourself with peaceful music, soft light, cozy blankets, and a lavender-scented eye pillow. Give yourself the gift of taking time to nurture your body, mind, and soul. You're definitely worth it.

"Silence is food for the soul...a wonderful place where wonderful things happen." — Barbara Berger, *A Road to Power*

❖ Sit up straight or lie comfortably on your back.

❖ Place your right hand over your heart and your left hand over your stomach just below the arc of your rib cage.

❖ Close your eyes and draw your attention inside.

❖ Take a deep breath, counting to four or five as you inhale and bringing your breath deeply into your lungs.

❖ Exhale gently for the same count, exhaling completely, then inhale to the same count again.

❖ Continue breathing, drawing an imaginary ribbon deep into your lungs as you inhale and exhaling it completely; this will help even out your breath.

❖ Consciously feel where your breath goes and draw it deeper into your body with each inhalation.

❖ Focus on your heart, gently creating space in your body; invite your breath to expand your ribs and lift your chest as you inhale.

❖ Maintain a straight spine and a spacious body as you exhale.

❖ With each inhalation, imagine drawing in soothing golden light. With each exhalation, breathe out tension and toxins, bringing your body into balance and harmony, your heart and mind into peace.

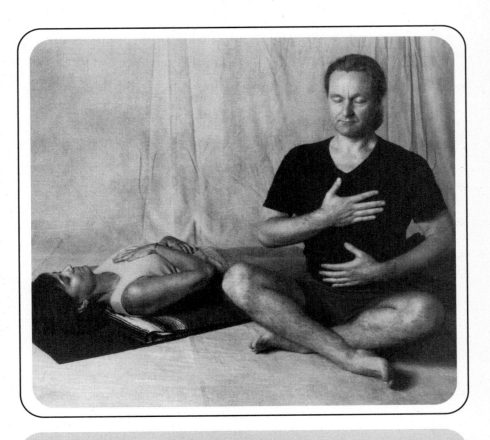

Benefits: Activates the parasympathetic nervous system, creating relaxation, centering, and calming. Lowers blood pressure, increases oxygenation throughout the body, and strengthens the respiratory system; detoxifies and cleanses the body.

"The main reason for healing is love." — Paracelsus

❖ Prepare a comfortable place for yourself on the floor and lie on your back.

❖ Place the soles of your feet together and draw your heels up toward your pelvis.

❖ With a blanket or pillow supporting each thigh, allow your knees to fall out to the sides.

❖ Place an eye pillow or soft cloth over your eyes.

❖ Bring your arms down to your sides, palms facing upward.

❖ Breathe deeply and consciously, feeling relaxation spread like a warm elixir throughout your body.

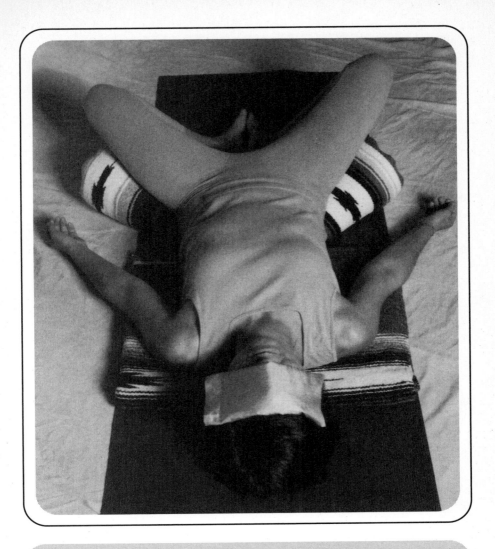

Benefits: Releases congestion in the pelvic area, relieves sciatica and lower back pain, and helps to prevent hernia and urinary problems; calms and relaxes the nervous system and lowers blood pressure.

"Seek not abroad, turn back into thyself for in the inner man dwells the Truth."
— St. Augustine

❖ Fold a blanket to fit the length of your torso and place the narrow end of it along the wall. Place another folded blanket or a pillow nearby.

❖ Sit sideways to the wall with your left hip as close to the wall as possible.

❖ Lean to your right side and swivel your hips to the left, bringing your buttocks as close to the wall as you can, then gently extend your legs up the wall (your knees may be bent for comfort).

❖ Lie on your back and, for support, place the extra blanket or pillow under your buttocks, hips, and lower back.

❖ Cover your eyes and let them rest gently in their sockets.

❖ Rest your arms on the floor slightly out from your sides, palms facing up, fingers relaxed.

❖ Relax. Breathe deeply a few times and allow your body to soften into the pose.

❖ To come out of the pose, bend your knees and roll onto your side. Take a few deep breaths, and then slowly unwind and raise yourself into a comfortable seated position.

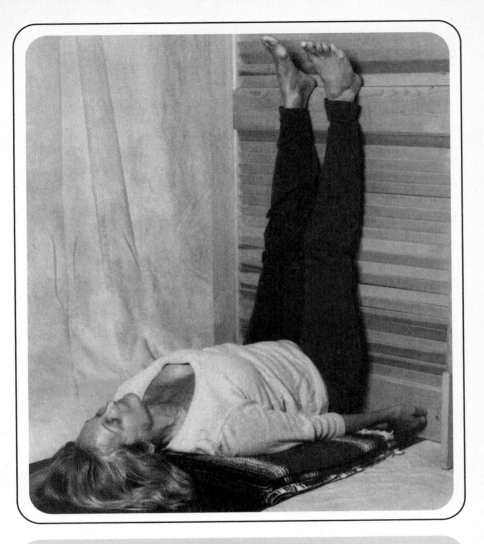

Benefits: Releases tension in the lower back and hips, helps to prevent varicose veins and swelling in the legs and feet, tones the abdominal organs, and relaxes the nervous system.

POSE 4: *Child's Pose*

"Supreme Bliss comes to the yogi whose mind is completely tranquil and whose passions are quieted."
— Bhagavad Gita

❖ Come onto your hands and knees, toes pointing back and the tops of your feet on the floor. Move your hips back and rest your buttocks on your heels.

❖ If you need support for your feet, you can place a blanket under your ankles.

❖ If you need support for your knees, you can place a blanket or pillow between your thighs and your calves.

❖ Soften your heart toward your thighs and bring your arms to rest, gently extended, with your elbows softly bent. Rest your forehead on the floor or turn your head to one side.

❖ You may place a pillow or blanket under your chest and/or head for comfort.

❖ As you inhale, feel your rib cage expand out to the sides, and as you exhale allow your body to release into the pose.

❖ Feel comforted and safe, like a nestled child.

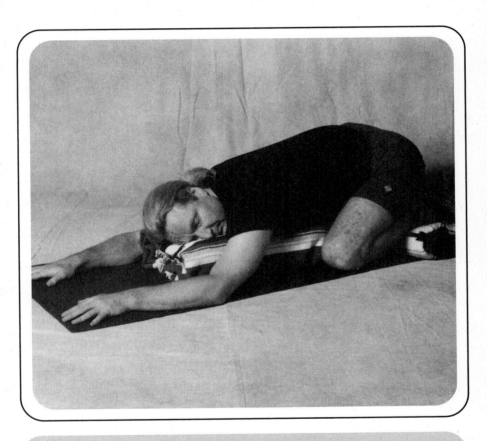

Benefits: A comfort pose, it takes strain off the lower back, cradles and softens the abdominal organs, relaxes the nervous system, encourages introspection, and creates a feeling of security and well-being.

"We realize that everything is a play of Consciousness and that, just as bubbles arise and subside in the ocean, whatever exists arises and subsides in the Self."
— Swami Muktananda

❖ Lie on your stomach, extend your legs, and separate them a comfortable distance apart, gently pointing your feet toward each other or straight back.

❖ Bring your arms forward and place your hands under your head with your forehead resting on them, or turn your head to one side for comfort.

❖ If you need support for your back, you may place a thin pillow under your belly and chest.

❖ Breathe deeply, all the way to your diaphragm, and feel your body release with each exhalation.

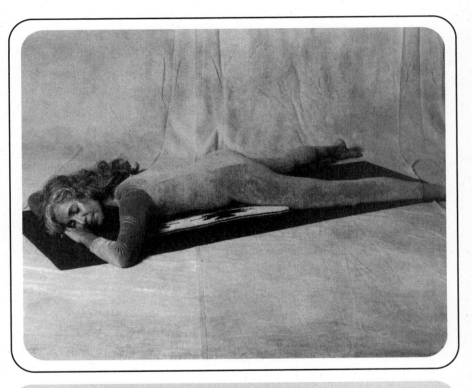

Benefits: Aids digestive and gastric problems;
releases the lower back and sacrum. Brings attention to the depth
of the breath and encourages diaphragmatic breathing.
Relaxes the abdominal area and expands the chest.

"There are many shifts occurring on many levels. These are the stirrings of the heart, and deeper, the Soul."

— Lyn Roberts-Herrick, *The Good Remembering*

❖ Lying on your back, place a blanket roll or pillow under your knees and an eye pillow or a soft cloth over your eyes.

❖ Let your arms rest on the floor slightly out from your sides, palms facing upward.

❖ Feel your shoulder blades and the back of your head resting gently against the floor. Scan your body and use your breath to release any tense areas.

❖ Expand any areas of tension with your breath as you inhale, and soften and release them as you exhale.

❖ Beginning with your feet, consciously relax. Continue to your calves, knees, and thighs. Relax your lower back and buttocks, ribs, shoulder blades, and so on, throughout your entire body.

❖ Let your eyeballs be suspended in their sockets and quiet your mind.

❖ Watch your breath. Let it flow effortlessly in and out.

❖ Withdraw your senses and enjoy the moment.

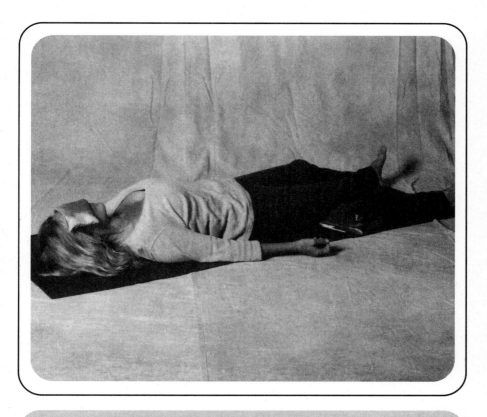

Benefits: Quiets and calms the mind and nervous system, relaxes and rejuvenates the body; this pose is a perfect remedy for the stresses of our fast-paced world.

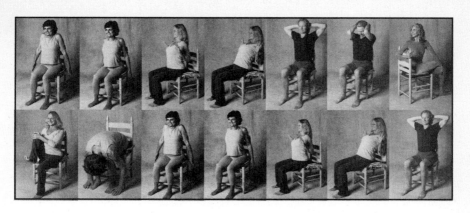

Sitting
Fit

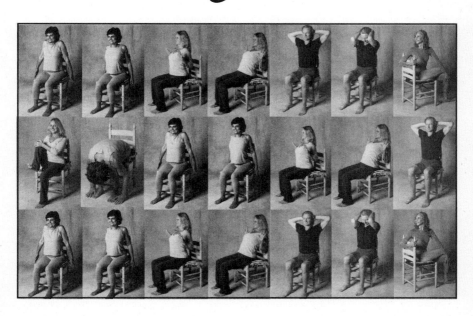

Do you work such long hours at your computer that you forget you have a body? Are you unable to get down and up off the floor? Haven't exercised or stretched for fifty years? No excuses! You can do yoga right where you're sitting: in your chair.

You can bring the benefits of the five-thousand-year-old body/mind wisdom of yoga into your twenty-first-century workplace and into your chair at home, work, or even on an airplane.

Integrating yoga into work time at your computer, or weaving it throughout your TV, telephone, and travel time, is a way to stretch, breathe, and relax throughout your day. You can be more centered, focused, and productive wherever you are.

Seated yoga can prevent and relieve stress, tension, and stiffness in your neck, back, and shoulders. It can ease backache, headache, carpal-tunnel problems, and problems associated with a sedentary lifestyle. It builds strength and flexibility, calms the nervous system, and soothes the soul.

Whether you're chained to a desk, recovering from surgery or illness, or have limited mobility for any reason, seated yoga will help you to live more comfortably in your body.

If you're breathing, you can do yoga. Conscious breathing (pranayama, or controlled breathing) is a good place to begin.

POSE 1: *Pranayama (Controlled Breathing)*

"You have to leave the city of your comfort and go into the wilderness of your intuition. What you'll discover will be wonderful. What you'll discover will be yourself."
— Alan Alda

Prana is the life force energy that animates all physical substance throughout the entire universe. It's the "stuff" the universe is made of. Einstein has shown us that everything is basically energy, and the ancient yogis knew that prana is that life force energy.

By learning to consciously bathe in and direct that energy within our bodies, we can gain more control over our bodies — and our minds.

Notice how your breathing pattern changes with excitement, anger, fear, or being hugged. We're usually not aware that our bodies hear and respond to everything we feel and think; if we're conscious of that interrelationship, we can control our bodies by controlling our minds. Breath and mind are intimately connected, so focusing the mind on the breath develops that awareness and control.

The practice of developing that sensitivity and skill is called "pranayama."

There are many variations and breathing techniques in pranayama. The pranayama practice described here is called *viloma*. It consists of a three-part breath, the inhalations and exhalations divided into thirds. The top-third breath extends from your upper chest to your breast line; the middle third, from your breast line to your waist; and the lower third, from your waist to your pubic bone.

CAUTION: *Those suffering from high blood pressure or heart problems should not hold their breath and should check with their doctor before doing this exercise.*

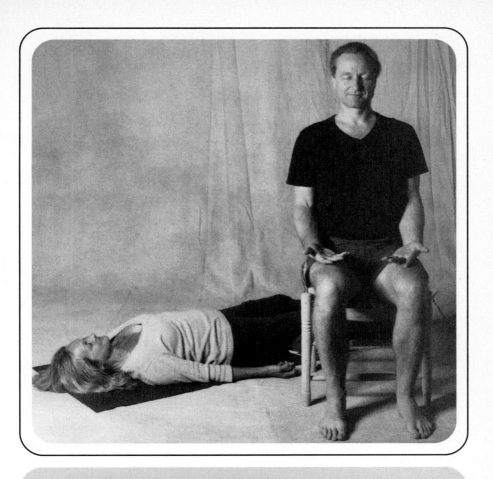

Benefits: Soothes the nervous system, oxygenates the lungs and bloodstream, lowers blood pressure, detoxifies the body, helps with insomnia, and calms the mind. Relieves stress, brings awareness and control to the body and peace and harmony to the spirit. Develops muscle control, increases lung capacity, and triggers the parasympathetic nervous system into the relaxation response.

If you are seated:

❖ Sit up straight with both feet flat on the floor, hip width apart.

❖ Open your arms out to your sides, with your palms facing outward.

❖ Feel your shoulder blades flatten against your back. Holding your shoulder blades right where they are, let your hands rest on the top of your thighs, palms facing up and fingers relaxed.

❖ Feel your heart lift and your head float upward.

If you are lying down:

❖ Check that your body is lying in a straight line and that you are comfortable.

❖ Place a pillow or rolled blanket under your knees, taking any pressure off your lower back.

❖ Place the back of your head on the floor in the same plane as your shoulders. Tip your chin up very slightly, opening your throat.

❖ Bring your arms out to your sides, palms facing up, and feel your shoulder blades flatten against your back.

❖ Holding your shoulder blades right where they are, bring your arms down to your sides, keeping your palms facing upward.

❖ Feel your heart space expand and your abdomen become more spacious.

❖ Close your eyes and draw your attention inside. Just be aware of your breathing rhythm for several moments.

❖ Inhale slowly and fully for a few breaths, building each breath and making it fuller than the previous one. Be sure to exhale slowly and completely; you can't inhale fully unless you totally exhale.

Viloma Inhaling

❖ As you inhale, fill the upper third of your body from your upper chest to your breast line and feel your breath expand your upper chest; pause for a heartbeat or two.

❖ Continue to inhale, expanding your lower rib cage and your waist. Pause.

❖ Continue your inhalation to fill your belly with your breath all the way down to your pubic bone. Pause and hold your breath for a couple of heartbeats.

❖ Exhale in one continuous flow of breath, slowly and with control. Take several deep, full breaths.

Viloma Exhaling

❖ Take a long, slow inhalation, filling your lungs completely.

❖ Exhale slowly, releasing the breath from your abdominal area, the lower third. Pause.

❖ Continue to exhale, releasing your midsection. Pause.

❖ Last, continue exhaling, releasing your breath from your upper chest. Pause and hold your breath for a heartbeat or two.

❖ Inhale deeply and slowly with one continuous breath. Take several breaths.

❖ Rest and repeat the sequence as many times as you feel is appropriate for you.

❖ You may find this challenging at first, but if you stay with it, you'll find that it becomes easier each time, and more rewarding.

POSE 2: *Shoulder Rolls*

"Do or do not. There is no try." — Yoda, *Star Wars*

❖ Sit up straight and inhale, drawing your shoulders up toward your ears.

❖ Inhale as you press your shoulder blades against your back and squeeze them tightly.

❖ Then press your shoulder blades toward each other, lifting your heart.

❖ Exhale and relax as you release your shoulder blades, sliding them down your back.

❖ Repeat three to five times.

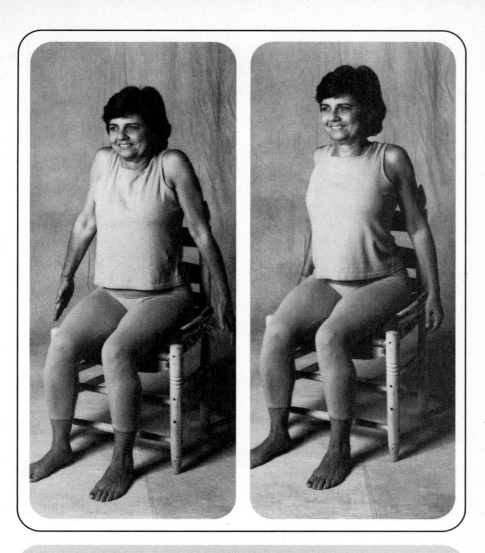

Benefits: Relaxes shoulder and neck tension, and increases
circulation to the head, neck, and shoulders.
Relieves headaches and releases upper back tightness.

"This above all: to thine own self be true, and it must follow as the night the day, Thou canst not then be false to any man."

— Shakespeare, *Hamlet*

- ❖ Sit up straight on the edge of your chair.

- ❖ Bend your elbows, press them back behind you and toward each other.

- ❖ Lift your heart as you inhale and press your elbows a bit closer together as you exhale.

- ❖ Lean back, keeping your back flat and heart lifted, and rest the back of your shoulders against your chair.

- ❖ Breathe deeply.

- ❖ Keeping your heart lifted and back flat, inhale as you sit up, leading with your heart.

- ❖ Repeat several times.

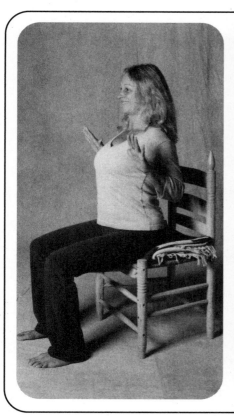 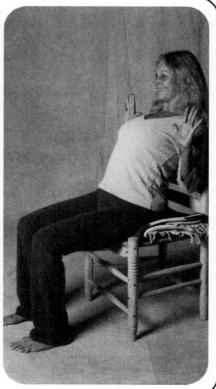

Benefits: Increases respiration. Flexes the spine. Relieves stiffness and relaxes the back, shoulders, and chest. Strengthens abdominal muscles and stimulates the endocrine system.

"One doesn't discover new lands without consenting to lose sight of the shore."
— André Gide

❖ Position yourself on the chair so that your feet are flat on the floor and your legs form a right angle between thighs and calves. You may need to sit toward the edge of your seat.

❖ Sit up straight and clasp your hands behind your head.

❖ Press your elbows back behind you and take a few deep breaths, lifting your heart.

❖ Lifting your ribs away from your hips, inhale and lengthen, creating space in your body.

❖ Keep your back flat and heart lifted as you exhale and drop your head forward, bringing your elbows toward each other.

❖ Tuck your chin in toward your throat and feel a nice, long stretch down the back of your neck and between your shoulder blades.

❖ Inhale and lengthen your spine as you sit up and open your elbows; exhale and drop your head forward again.

❖ Repeat five times.

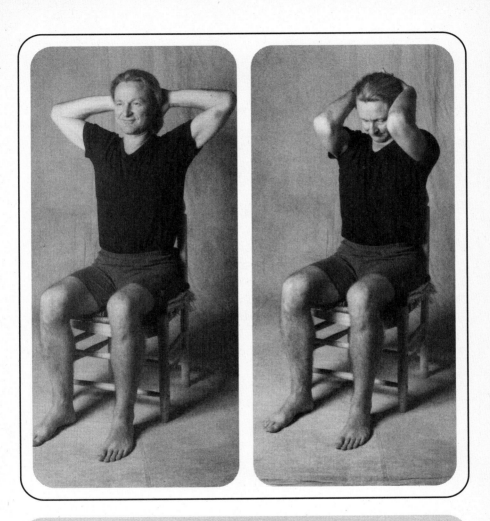

Benefits: Stretches the back of the neck, spine, rib cage, and arms. Deepens respiration and massages internal organs. Releases tension, relieves headache, stimulates the thyroid, and massages the lymph glands.

"Here's the test to find whether your mission on earth is finished. If you're alive, it isn't."
— Richard Bach

❖ Sit up straight toward the edge of your seat.

❖ Cross your right leg over your left.

❖ Place your left hand on the inside of your left knee.

❖ Inhale deeply as you lengthen through the crown of your head.

❖ Exhale as you twist to the right, bringing your right elbow or shoulder around toward the back of your chair.

❖ Take three to five full breaths. Lift through the crown of your head as you inhale and twist a little deeper as you exhale.

❖ To release the pose, keep lengthening your spine and come back to center as you exhale.

❖ Repeat for three to five breaths, then twist on the other side.

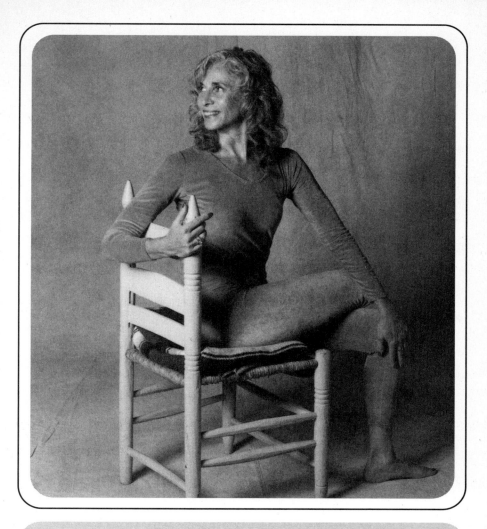

Benefits: Massages organs of digestion and elimination, relieving constipation and indigestion; releases back strain and tension and relaxes the nervous system. Creates flexibility in the spine, hydrates the disks, and circulates cerebrospinal fluid.

POSE 6: *Hamstring Stretch*

"My philosophy is that not only are you responsible for your life, but doing the best at this moment. That puts you in the best place for the next moment."
— Oprah Winfrey

❖ Sitting on the edge of your seat, bring both feet flat on the floor with your ankles directly under your knees.

❖ Flatten your shoulder blades against your back and keep your heart lifted as you raise your right knee and clasp it with both hands.

❖ Draw your knee in toward your rib cage and bring your lower ribs up and toward your right thigh, keeping your back flat and chest lifted.

❖ Breathe deeply for three to five breaths.

❖ Release and stretch the other side.

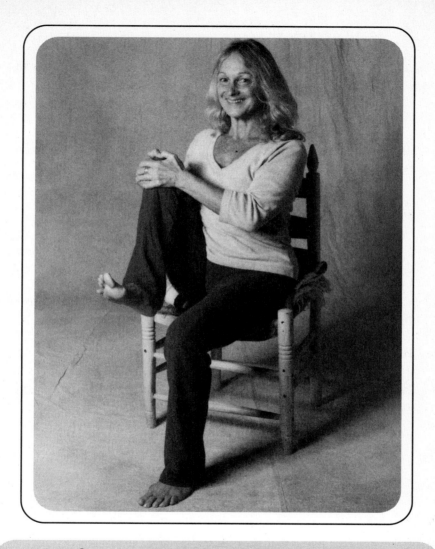

Benefits: Stretches hamstrings, releasing lower-back tension; massages abdominal area, relieving constipation, bloating, and indigestion. Strengthens back and abdominal area.

POSE 7: *Half Forward Fold*

"You gain strength, courage, and confidence by every experience in which you really stop to look fear in the face. You must do the thing you think you cannot do."
— Eleanor Roosevelt

❖ Sitting with your tailbone against the back of your seat, lengthen your spine as you lift through the crown of your head.

❖ Interlace your fingers and place your hands behind your head, elbows back.

❖ Inhale as you lean forward from the hips, leading with your heart. Keep your elbows back, your back flat, and chin up.

❖ If you can bend all the way forward, relax your chest onto your thighs and let your arms release down beside your legs.

❖ Breathe deeply for three to five breaths.

❖ Replace your hands on the back of your head and sit up, keeping your elbows pressing back and your heart lifting.

❖ Repeat three times.

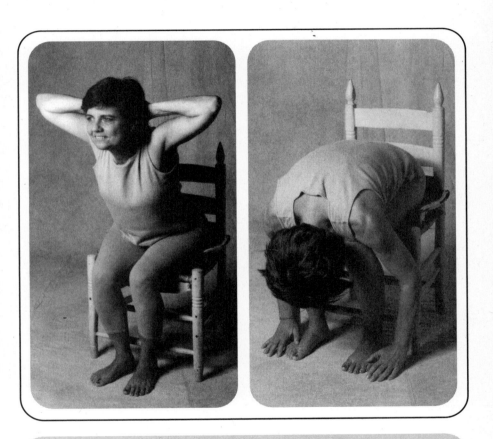

Benefits: Builds strength in the back and releases tension in the neck. Stimulates respiration, stretches the arms, back, and the front of the body.

Barnard, Neal. *Food for Life.* New York: Harmony Books, 1993.

Bell, Lorna, and Eudora Seyfer. *Gentle Yoga.* Berkeley: Celestial Arts, 1982.

Chopra, Deepak. *Ageless Body, Timeless Mind: The Quantum Alternative to Growing Old.* New York: Harmony Books, 1993.

Devi, Nischala. *The Healing Path of Yoga.* New York: Three Rivers Press, 2000.

Francina, Suza. *The New Yoga for People over 50.* Deerfield Beach, Fla.: Health Communications, 1997.

Hewitt, James. *The Complete Yoga Book.* New York: Schocken Books, 1977.

Iyengar, B. K. S. *Light on Yoga.* New York: Schocken Books, 1966.

Kravette, Stephen. *Alternatives to Aging.* West Chester, Pa.: Whitford Press, 1989.

Lusk, Julie T. *Desktop Yoga.* New York: Penguin/Putnam, 1998.

Null, Gary. *Reverse the Aging Process Naturally.* New York: Villard Books/Random House, 1993.

Ornish, Dean. *Reversing Heart Disease.* New York: Random House, 1990.

Paul, Stephen C. *Inneractions.* New York: HarperCollins, 1992.

Robbins, John. *Diet for a New America.* Novato, Calif.: H J Kramer, 1987.

Samskrti and Veda. *Hatha Yoga, Manual I.* Honesdale, Pa.: The Himalayan International Institute of Yoga Science and Philosophy, 1977.

Scaravelli, Vanda. *Awakening the Spine.* San Francisco: HarperSanFrancisco, 1991.

Trager, Milton. *Trager Mentastics.* Barrytown, N.Y.: Station Hill Press, 1987.

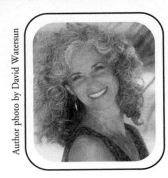

Author photo by David Watersun

Susan Winter Ward is an internationally recognized yoga instructor, author, and video producer. She is the founder of Yoga for the Young at Heart™, a multimedia publisher that creates an informative and inspiring collection of CD-ROMs, videos, audio tapes, books, and television programs, as well as exciting vacation retreats.

Susan began practicing yoga in 1990 at White Lotus Foundation in Santa Barbara, California. She was led to yoga in her search for relief from ten years of back pain and was so impressed with the results that within two years, she became a teacher so she could share the blessings of yoga. Teaching mostly seniors and beginners, Susan has developed a gentle and encouraging teaching approach based on the vinyasa-style White Lotus Flow Series and is now strongly influenced by John Friend's heart-centered Anusara Yoga. Anusara's principles of alignment and the concept of honoring the body's innate intelligence form an integral foundation for Susan's teaching.

Susan leads her unique yoga classes and workshops at retreats and conferences worldwide. She has led classes at the National Institute for the Clinical Application of Behavioral Medicine, the International Conference on Business and Consciousness, the South West Yoga Conference, Inner Voyage cruises and events, International Innate Intelligence (Network Spinal Analysis) Transformational Gate Intensives, Whole Life, and other expos. She also serves on the teaching staff and board of directors of the American Yoga College and was a member of the teaching faculty of Deepak Chopra's Web site, MyPotential.com.

She has written articles for a variety of national magazines and newspapers and her television series, *Yoga for the Young at Heart,* currently airs in Santa Fe, New Mexico.

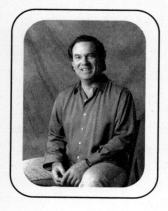

John Sirois began photographing people when he was eight, using his treasured Kodak Brownie Hawkeye to photograph his ten siblings. He still enjoys photographing people, and he has found that viewing a photograph has more impact on a person's self-perception than looking in a mirror. Originally from Massachusetts, John now resides in Santa Barbara, California.

Yoga for the Young at Heart Products

CD-ROM

Sitting Fit Anytime: Interactive CD-ROM & ScreenSaver
$34.95 • ISBN 0-9651409-6-2
Designed to remind you that you have a body while working at your computer, this screen saver will help you relieve tension, release stress, and re-energize right where you sit.

Videos

Yoga for the Young at Heart: The Original Program
50 minutes • $19.95 • ISBN: 0-9651409-2-X
A class designed especially for seniors and less flexible beginners of all ages.

Embracing Menopause: A Path to Peace and Power
58 minutes • $19.95 • ISBN: 0-9651409-3-8
A flowing yoga class designed to acknowledge and create balance in harmony with the natural menopause process.

Sitting Fit Anytime: Easy & Effective Chair Yoga
43 minutes • $19.95 • ISBN 0-9651409-5-4
Ideal for the desk-bound, those in rehabilitation, and the physically challenged.

Audiotapes

Joy of Rejuvenation
60 minutes • $9.95 • ISBN: 0-9651409-0-3
A simple, effective, and clearly guided one-hour yoga class with peaceful Native American flute music accompaniment.

Sitting Fit: Yoga Bits
60 minutes • $9.95 • ISBN: 0-9651409-1-1
Chosen for use in-flight by Delta Airlines, this tape offers a convenient seated yoga program of four 15-minute mini classes.

For more information or to place an order call Yoga for the Young at Heart at:
Post Office Box 2228, Pagosa Springs, Colorado 81147
Phone: 800-558-9642 or 970-731-YOGA (9642)
Fax: 970-731-9510 • Web site: www.yogaheart.com

Models

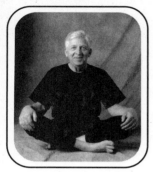

Otto Mortensen, an architect, came to America from Copenhagen in 1957. He has been a yoga enthusiast for more than twenty years.

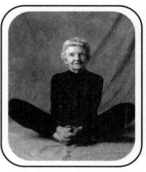

Babs Raymond joined Susan's yoga class in 1993. Although she is blind, she found the practice of yoga accessible and describes Susan's class as "entirely uplifting."

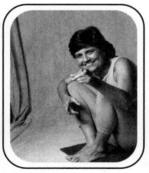

Star Riparetti took Susan to her first yoga class. She is owner of Star Essence, producing flower and gemstone essences, and leads spiritual adventures to Peru.

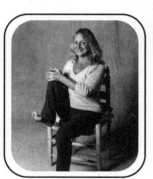

Anita Stith is co-owner of a yoga studio in Santa Barbara, California, where she teaches. She also teaches yoga at senior centers and to mentally and physically challenged students.

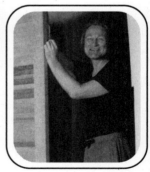

Karl Schiffmann teaches yoga at the Santa Barbara Yoga Center. He is also a musician and leads salsa dance retreats.

Nataraj Publishing, a division of
New World Library, is dedicated to
publishing books and cassettes that inspire
and challenge us to improve the quality
of our lives and our world.
Our books and cassettes are available
at bookstores everywhere.
For a complete catalog, contact:

New World Library
14 Pamaron Way
Novato, California 94949

Phone: (415) 884-2100
Fax: (415) 884-2199
Or call toll free: (800) 972-6657
Catalog requests: Ext. 50
Ordering: Ext. 52

E-mail: escort@nwlib.com
www.newworldlibrary.com